Monitoring Tissue Perfusion and Oxygenation

Editors

SHANNAN K. HAMLIN
C. LEE PARMLEY

CRITICAL CARE NURSING CLINICS OF NORTH AMERICA

www.ccnursing.theclinics.com

Consulting Editor
JAN FOSTER

September 2014 • Volume 26 • Number 3

ELSEVIER

1600 John F. Kennedy Boulevard • Suite 1800 • Philadelphia, Pennsylvania, 19103-2899

http://www.theclinics.com

CRITICAL CARE NURSING CLINICS OF NORTH AMERICA Volume 26, Number 3
September 2014 ISSN 0899-5885, ISBN-13: 978-0-323-32319-2

Editor: Kerry Holland
Developmental Editor: Stephanie Carter

Critical Care Nursing Clinics of North America (ISSN 0899-5885) is published quarterly by Elsevier Inc., 360 Park Avenue South, New York, NY 10010-1710. Months of issue are March, June, September, and December. Business and Editorial Offices: 1600 John F. Kennedy Blvd., Suite 1800, Philadelphia, PA 19103-2899. Periodicals postage paid at New York, NY and additional mailing offices. Subscription prices are $150.00 per year for US individuals, $328.00 per year for US institutions, $80.00 per year for US students and residents, $200.00 per year for Canadian individuals, $412.00 per year for Canadian institutions, $230.00 per year for international individuals, $412.00 per year for international institutions and $115.00 per year for Canadian and international students/residents. To receive student/resident rate, orders must be accompanied by name of affiliated institution, data of term, and the *signature* of program/residency coordinator on institution letterhead. Orders will be billed at individual rate until proof of status is received. Foreign air speed delivery is included in all *Clinics* subscription prices. All prices are subject to change without notice. **POSTMASTER:** Send address changes to *Critical Care Nursing Clinics of North America*, Elsevier Health Sciences Division, Subscription Customer Service, 3251 Riverport Lane, Maryland Heights, MO 63043. **Customer Service: 1-800-654-2452 (US and Canada); 314-447-8871 (outside US and Canada). Fax: 314-447-8029. E-mail: JournalsCustomerService-usa@elsevier.com (for print support) and JournalsOnlineSupport-usa@elsevier.com (for online support).**

Reprints. For copies of 100 or more of articles in this publication, please contact the Commercial Reprints Department, Elsevier Inc., 360 Park Avenue South, New York, New York, 10010-1710; Tel.: 212-633-3874, Fax: 212-633-3820, and E-mail: reprints@elsevier.com.

Critical Care Nursing Clinics of North America is covered in *MEDLINE/PubMed (Index Medicus), International Nursing Index, Nursing Citation Index, Cumulative Index to Nursing and Allied Health Literature, and RNdex Top 100.*

Contributors

CONSULTING EDITOR

JAN FOSTER, PhD, RN, CNS
College of Nursing, Texas Woman's University, Houston, Texas

EDITORS

SHANNAN K. HAMLIN, PhD, RN, ACNP-BC, AGACNP-BC, CCRN
Program Director, Nursing Research and Evidence-Based Practice, Houston Methodist Hospital, Houston, Texas

C. LEE PARMLEY, MD, JD, MMHC
Chief of Staff, Executive Medical Director for Critical Care, Vanderbilt University Hospital; Professor, Department of Anesthesiology, Critical Care Division, Vanderbilt University School of Medicine, Nashville, Tennessee

AUTHORS

DANIEL L. ARELLANO, MSN, RN, ACNP-BC, CCRN, CEN
Critical Care Nurse Practitioner, Division of Critical Care, Department of Medicine, Houston Methodist Hospital; Instructor of Nursing; Department of Family Health, School of Nursing, University of Texas Health Science Center at Houston, Houston, Texas

NATHAN ASHBY, MD
Assistant Professor of Anesthesiology/Critical Care Medicine and Adjunct Assistant Professor of Nursing, Division of Anesthesiology Critical Care Medicine, Vanderbilt University Medical Center, Nashville, Tennessee

PENELOPE S. BENEDIK, PhD, RN, CRNA, RRT
Associate Professor of Clinical Nursing, Department of Acute and Continuing Care, School of Nursing, Division of Nurse Anesthesia, University of Texas Health Science Center at Houston, Houston, Texas

KRISTI CUSTARD, BSN, RN
Assistant Nurse Manager, Cardiovascular Recovery Room, Baylor St. Luke's Medical Center, Houston, Texas

SHANNAN K. HAMLIN, PhD, RN, ACNP-BC, AGACNP-BC, CCRN
Program Director, Nursing Research and Evidence-Based Practice, Houston Methodist Hospital, Houston, Texas

SANDRA K. HANNEMAN, PhD, RN, FAAN
Jerold B. Katz Distinguished Professor for Nursing Research, Center for Nursing Research, School of Nursing, University of Texas Health Science Center at Houston, Houston, Texas

ALEXANDER JOHNSON, MSN, RN, ACNP-BC, CCNS, CCRN
Clinical Nurse Specialist for Critical Care, Central DuPage Hospital, Cadence Health, Winfield, Illinois

LAURA L. LIPP, MS, APRN, ACNP-BC, CNRN
Acute Care Nurse Practitioner, Nurse Practitioner Service, Houston Methodist Hospital, Houston, Texas

MEHR MOHAJER-ESFAHANI, BSN, RN
Associate Manager for Critical Care, Central DuPage Hospital, Cadence Health, Winfield, Illinois

C. LEE PARMLEY, MD, JD, MMHC
Chief of Staff, Executive Medical Director for Critical Care, Vanderbilt University Hospital; Professor, Department of Anesthesiology, Critical Care Division, Vanderbilt University School of Medicine, Nashville, Tennessee

CLAUDIA DISABATINO SMITH, PhD, RN, NE-BC
Director of Nursing Research, Baylor St. Luke's Medical Center, Houston, Texas

JOSHUA SQUIERS, PhD, ACNP
Assistant Professor of Nursing and Anesthesiology/Critical Care Medicine, Vanderbilt University School of Nursing, Nashville, Tennessee

Contents

Preface: Monitoring Tissue Perfusion and Oxygenation

ix

Shannan K. Hamlin and C. Lee Parmley

A Historical Perspective on the Development of Modern Concepts of Tissue Perfusion: Prehistory to the Twentieth Century

297

Nathan Ashby and Joshua Squiers

The historical development of the concept of perfusion is traced, with particular focus on the development of the modern clinical concepts of perfusion through the fields of anatomy, physiology, and biochemistry. This article reviews many of the significant contributors to the changing ideas of perfusion up through the twentieth century that have influenced the modern physiologic circulatory and metabolic models. The developments outlined have provided the modern model of perfusion, linking the cardiopulmonary circulation, tissue oxygen utilization and carbon dioxide production, food intake, tissue waste production and elimination, and ultimately the production and utilization of ATP in the body.

Microcirculatory Oxygen Transport and Utilization

311

Shannan K. Hamlin, C. Lee Parmley, and Sandra K. Hanneman

The cardiovascular system (macrocirculation) circulates blood throughout the body, but the microcirculation is responsible for modifying tissue perfusion and adapting it to metabolic demand. Hemodynamic assessment and monitoring of the critically ill patient is typically focused on global measures of oxygen transport and utilization, which do not evaluate the status of the microcirculation. Despite achievement and maintenance of global hemodynamic and oxygenation goals, patients may develop microcirculatory dysfunction with associated organ failure. A thorough understanding of the microcirculatory system under physiologic conditions will assist the clinician in early recognition of microcirculatory dysfunction in impending and actual disease states.

The Physiologic Role of Erythrocytes in Oxygen Delivery and Implications for Blood Storage

325

Penelope S. Benedik and Shannan K. Hamlin

Erythrocytes are not just oxygen delivery devices but play an active metabolic role in modulating microvascular blood flow. Hemoglobin and red blood cell morphology change as local oxygen levels fall, eliciting the release of adenosine triphosphate and nitric oxide to initiate local vasodilation. Aged erythrocytes undergo physical and functional changes such that some of the red cell's most physiologically helpful attributes are diminished. This article reviews the functional anatomy and applied physiology of the erythrocyte and the microcirculation with an emphasis on how erythrocytes modulate microvascular function. The effects of cell storage on the metabolic functions of the erythrocyte are also briefly discussed.

Basic Concepts of Hemorheology in Microvascular Hemodynamics   337

Shannan K. Hamlin and Penelope S. Benedik

> Blood rheology, or hemorheology, involves the flow and deformation behavior of blood and its formed elements (ie, erythrocytes, leukocytes, platelets). The adequacy of blood flow to meet metabolic demands through large circulatory vessels depends highly on vascular control mechanisms. However, the extent to which rheologic properties of blood contribute to vascular flow resistance, particularly in the microcirculation, is becoming more appreciated. Current evidence suggests that microvascular blood flow is determined by local vessel resistance and hemorheologic factors such as blood viscosity, erythrocyte deformability, and erythrocyte aggregation. Such knowledge will aid clinicians caring for patients with hemodynamic alterations.

Monitoring Tissue Blood Flow and Oxygenation: A Brief Review of Emerging Techniques   345

Penelope S. Benedik

> This article describes promising emerging technologies developed for measuring tissue-level oxygenation or perfusion, each with its own inherent limitations. The end user must understand what the instrument measures and how to interpret the readings. Optical monitoring using near-infrared spectrometry, Doppler shift, and videomicroscopy are discussed in terms of their application at the tissue level. Assessment of the metabolic state of the extracellular space with existing technology and proxy indicators of metabolic status are discussed. Also addressed are potential sources of variation for each technique, and the role that the clinician plays in the proper interpretation of the data.

Exploring Hemodynamics: A Review of Current and Emerging Noninvasive Monitoring Techniques   357

Alexander Johnson and Mehr Mohajer-Esfahani

> The lack of randomized controlled trials suggesting improved outcomes with pulmonary artery catheter use and pressure-based hemodynamic monitoring has led to a decrease in pulmonary artery catheter use. However, an increasing amount of literature supporting stroke volume optimization (SVO) has caused a paradigm shift from pressure-based to flow-based techniques. This article discusses emerging flow-based techniques, supporting evidence, and considerations for use in critical care for methods such as Doppler, pulse contour, bioimpedance, bioreactance, and exhaled carbon dioxide. Regardless of the device chosen, the SVO algorithm approach should be considered, and volume challenges should be guided by dynamic assessments of fluid responsiveness.

The Experience of Family Members of ICU Patients Who Require Extensive Monitoring: A Qualitative Study   377

Claudia DiSabatino Smith and Kristi Custard

> A mixed methods study using family research with a phenomenological approach (n = 5 families) was conducted to explore family members' perceptions about the extensive monitoring technology used on their critically

ill family member after cardiac surgery, as experienced when family members initially visited the patient in the cardiovascular intensive care unit. Five relevant themes emerged: overwhelmed by all of the machines; feelings of uncertainty; methods of coping; meaning of the numbers on the machines; and need for education.

Brain Perfusion and Oxygenation   389

Laura L. Lipp

Maintenance of brain perfusion and oxygenation is of paramount importance to patient outcome with various types of brain injuries (traumatic, ischemic, and hemorrhagic). Historically, monitoring of intracranial pressure and cerebral perfusion pressure has been the mainstay of neuromonitoring techniques used at the critical care bedside to monitor brain perfusion and oxygenation. This article describes the bedside neuromonitoring techniques that have emerged for use with these patients in the critical care area. To give the reader an understanding of the functionality of these neuromonitoring techniques, the article first summarizes the physiology of brain perfusion and oxygenation.

Microcirculatory Alterations in Shock States   399

Shannan K. Hamlin, C. Lee Parmley, and Sandra K. Hanneman

Functional components of the microcirculation provide oxygen and nutrients and remove waste products from the tissue beds of the body's organs. Shock states overwhelmingly stress functional capacity of the microcirculation, resulting in microcirculatory failure. In septic shock, inflammatory mediators contribute to hemodynamic instability. In nonseptic shock states, the microcirculation is better able to compensate for alterations in vascular resistance, cardiac output, and blood pressure. Therefore, global hemodynamic and oxygen delivery parameters are appropriate for assessing, monitoring, and guiding therapy in hypovolemic and cardiogenic shock but, alone, are inadequate for septic shock.

Vasopressor Weaning in Patients with Septic Shock   413

Daniel L. Arellano and Sandra K. Hanneman

The purpose of this article is to propose optimal weaning of vasopressors in patients with septic shock. Topics discussed include pathophysiology of sepsis and septic shock, treatment guidelines for sepsis, autoregulation of blood flow, vasopressors used in septic shock, weaning recommendations, monitor alarms in the intensive care unit, and new directions in sepsis research.

Index   427

Monitoring Tissue Perfusion and Oxygenation

CRITICAL CARE NURSING
CLINICS OF NORTH AMERICA

FORTHCOMING ISSUES

December 2014
Quality
Bobbi Leeper and Rosemary Luquire, *Editors*

March 2015
Certified Registered Nurse Anesthesia:
Critical Care Nursing in the Operating Room
Holly Robins and
Stanley H. Rosenbaum, *Editors*

June 2015
Violence, War, and Traumatic Injury
Karen Bergman, *Editor*

RECENT ISSUES

June 2014
Nutrition in Critical Illness
Miranda K. Kelly and Jody Collins, *Editors*

March 2014
Aging and Critical Care
Sonya R. Hardin, *Editor*

December 2013
Hematology
Mary Lou Warren and Melissa McLenon,
Editors

NOW AVAILABLE FOR YOUR iPhone and iPad

Preface

Monitoring Tissue Perfusion and Oxygenation

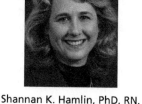

Shannan K. Hamlin, PhD, RN, ACNP-BC, AGACNP-BC, CCRN

C. Lee Parmley, MD, JD, MMHC

Editors

The concept of tissue perfusion and cellular oxygenation involves a fine-tuned interaction between anatomic, physiologic, and biochemical processes. These processes work to ensure oxygen delivery meets or exceeds cellular oxygen demand. The competence with which these processes occur is critical to organ functioning and ultimately determines patient survival. To estimate the adequacy of tissue perfusion, clinicians caring for critically ill patients have relied on macrovascular indices such as blood pressure and cardiac output to monitor organ perfusion. Evidence produced over the last decade has clearly shown that the microvasculature is the critical region responsible for meeting the metabolic oxygen demands of the tissues by actively and passively regulating the distribution of red blood cells and plasma throughout individual organs. Monitoring the state of the microvasculature, however, remains problematic as bedside techniques have not kept up with the pace of microvascular knowledge acquisition in the area of tissue perfusion. The concepts presented in this special issue are complex, leaving many to argue they are out of the bedside clinicians' required scope of knowledge. The authors of this collective body of work will counter that it is imperative for clinicians to expand their knowledge beyond that of a purely macrovascular understanding and to appreciate the complex intermingling of the microvasculature and macrovasculature.

Critical care clinicians must be knowledgeable about the anatomic, physiologic, and biochemical processes that are critical to the restoration of a functioning microvascular affecting organ perfusion. These basic physiologic processes critical to tissue perfusion and cellular oxygenation are presented in this issue of *Critical Care Nursing Clinics of North America* on "Monitoring Tissue Perfusion and Oxygenation." A working knowledge of oxygen delivery and oxygen consumption at the microvascular level will provide critical information needed for clinicians to continuously question the adequacy of tissue perfusion given our current lack of microvascular bedside monitoring

Crit Care Nurs Clin N Am 26 (2014) ix–x
http://dx.doi.org/10.1016/j.ccell.2014.05.002
0899-5885/14/$ – see front matter © 2014 Elsevier Inc. All rights reserved.

ccnursing.theclinics.com

techniques. The authors of this special issue have strived to broaden the readers' knowledge and understanding that despite what may look to be a hemodynamically stable patient, an altered microvasculature may be undermining the patient's ability to restore organ functioning.

The first article will take the reader back to our roots of tissue perfusion understanding and present an account through time of significant contributors to changing thoughts and ideas that have influenced our modern understanding of physiologic circulatory and metabolic models. The next three articles provide a basic understanding of microvascular oxygen transport and utilization in physiologic states. The important role of the erythrocyte in oxygen delivery is highlighted along with blood flow behavior as it relates to the erythrocyte. Having a base knowledge of physiologic tissue perfusion and cellular oxygenation concepts allows a better understanding of alterations in blood flow and oxygenation.

The next three articles found in this special issue focus on tissue blood flow and oxygenation monitoring techniques, including noninvasive monitoring, which has evolved over the last 15 years to become a more accurate and precise method for monitoring tissue perfusion. The patient's family perspective concerning extensive hemodynamic monitoring is presented as a qualitative study in the next article. As clinicians are focused more on patient-centered and family-centered care, the perspective of the family who experience their loved one connected to extensive high-tech monitoring can have significant implications for family coping and the added need for improved family education surrounding the intensive care unit environment.

The final three articles highlight tissue perfusion and oxygenation abnormalities in patients with brain injury and shock states. The final article in our series addresses a common question of how best to wean vasopressors in patients with septic shock, providing evidence-based recommendations.

Each of the articles presented in this special issue provides important information to the care of critically ill patients. A paradigm shift now focuses our attention on the microvasculature as the center of organ dysfunction and failure. As such, critical care clinicians should be wary of microvascular perfusion and consider microcirculation dysfunction when global hemodynamic parameters suggest a stable macrocirulation despite persistent organ function decline. Perhaps in the near future we can anticipate newer bedside technologies that will better monitor the state of microvascular perfusion and cellular oxygenation.

Shannan K. Hamlin, PhD, RN, ACNP-BC, AGACNP-BC, CCRN
Houston Methodist Hospital
MGJ 11-017
Houston, TX 77030, USA

C. Lee Parmley, MD, JD, MMHC
Vanderbilt University Hospital
1211 21st Avenue South, S3408 MCN
Nashville, TN 37212, USA

E-mail addresses:
SHamlin@HoustonMethodist.org (S.K. Hamlin)
Clifford.L.Parmley@Vanderbilt.Edu (C.L. Parmley)

A Historical Perspective on the Development of Modern Concepts of Tissue Perfusion

Prehistory to the Twentieth Century

Nathan Ashby, MD[a],*, Joshua Squiers, PhD, ACNP[b]

KEYWORDS

- History • Perfusion • Physiology

KEY POINTS

- The modern concept of perfusion encompasses a variety of anatomic, physiologic, and biochemical ideas. These are incorporated into a model of how the body delivers fuel substrates and oxygen to target tissues for their conversion into energy that the body uses for the biochemical processes of life and how the body removes the waste byproducts that occur during these biochemical processes.
- The modern concept of perfusion has largely grown out of discoveries that have taken centuries of scientific inquiry.
- The concept of tissue perfusion continues to evolve and develop.
- Although the basic groundwork of tissue perfusion was completed by the middle of the twentieth century, there continue to be discoveries and refinements of understanding. As the means of exploring the intracellular milieu improve, additional links become apparent.
- These new discoveries are also opening the door to new ways to bring theoretic knowledge to bedside monitoring and care.

INTRODUCTION

Few processes are more basic to life than the delivery of oxygen and nutrients to cells and the removal of carbon dioxide and waste products from them. Without these functions, cellular metabolism and work stop and the cell dies (or must go into a state of

Conflict of Interest: Nil.
[a] Division of Anesthesiology Critical Care Medicine, Vanderbilt University Medical Center, 526 MAB, 1211 Medical Center Drive, Nashville, TN 37232, USA; [b] Vanderbilt University School of Nursing, Frist Hall 338, 461 21st Avenue South, Nashville, TN 37240, USA
* Corresponding author.
E-mail address: nathan.ashby@vanderbilt.edu

suspended animation). In single-celled organisms, these actions are accomplished through direct contact with the environment. In more complex organisms, these fundamental activities become significantly more complex. Multiple cell types with specific functions and arranged in specific positions move the necessary metabolic substrates from the external environment to the internal one. Once internalized, the substrates are distributed according to the utilization of the target cells. Yet despite this complex system, the basic nature of the process remains: deliver oxygen and nutrients while removing toxic metabolic byproducts. Given the importance of this process in mammalian biology, it is remarkable how difficult the concept of perfusion has been for the medical sciences to unravel and understand.

The origins of the concepts that eventually formed the current understanding of perfusion are convoluted. The fundamentals of circulation have been discovered and rediscovered and arranged and rearranged until finally placed in a formal framework in the 1600s. Once a formal understanding of the circulatory system became more widely accepted and agreed on, a series of ever more complicated pieces of the puzzle layered on one another until modern times. Tissue perfusion is now viewed as a web of anatomy, physiology, and biochemistry. So fundamental a topic to mammalian biology and medicine as tissue perfusion would be thought firmly quantified and conceptualized by the time of modern medical science. Understanding of what happens at the cellular level, however, continues to evolve to this day. The purpose of this article is to trace some of the important discoveries, and the people responsible for them, that have led to the modern concept of tissue perfusion.

ANATOMIC ERA

The concept of perfusion is one that has developed over centuries rather than the relatively brief time frame of scientific discoveries, such as DNA (**Table 1**). For millennia, there was no formal and systematic concept of the inner workings of the body. In order for the concept of tissue perfusion to reach its current state, a basic understanding of the functional anatomy, and circulation in particular, of the human body was needed.

Evidence exists that ancient humans had a basic understanding of the circulatory system. In a review of the early history of the circulatory system, Garrison[1] points out that cave paintings show the importance of striking the heart in ending the life of wild game. Garrison also notes that early man recognized that compressing the carotids led to a loss of consciousness and that staunching the flow of blood was key in preventing death from wounds on the battlefield.[1] He also notes that certain cultures recognized that the beating heart of a sacrificial victim embodied the life of the victim being sacrificed to the gods. Yet, even with this knowledge of what has been termed, *anatomic instinct*,[1] the anatomy and physiology of the circulatory system took centuries to understand, formalize, and elucidate.

The understanding of which organs were involved in circulation and how they were connected stymied early thinkers. For much of the time that man has walked the Earth, there was neither time nor excess resources to devote to formalized scientific inquiry. With the development of more complex cultures, time and resources became available to expend on scientific inquiries beyond the focus on basic subsistence. Art, music, and science all began to grow and develop. Early scientific understandings of the circulatory system begin to appear in this time frame (1000–500 BC). Although many historians of medicine point to the Greek system as the foundation of modern circulation, with Hippocrates the most recognized early source,[2] similar developments were occurring in other advancing societies at the time. Some researchers point to early Chinese texts as the earliest written evidence of the concept of circulation of

Table 1 General periods of historical development	
Anatomic period	
Prehistory–1000 BC	"Anatomic instinct"
1000 BC–500 BC	Early inquiry in multiple civilizations
500 BC–200 BC	Development of Greek humoral theories
200 BC–100 AD	No advances, Greek theories persist
100 AD–200 AD	Development of galenic theories
200 AD–1400s AD	No significant advances in the West, galenic principles persist
850 AD–1200s AD	Arabic refinement of galenic anatomy and principles
1200 AD–1500 AD	Arabic challenges to galenic anatomy and principles
1400s AD–1600s AD	Western challenges to galenic anatomy
1628 AD	Publication of *Exercitatio Anatomica de Motu Cordis et Sanguinis in Animalibus* by William Harvey
1600s AD–1700s AD	Description of microscopic anatomy
Physiology and biochemistry era	
1770s AD	Discovery of oxygen
1783 AD	Discovery of role of oxygen in metabolism
1840 AD	Discovery of hemoglobin
1899 AD	Discovery of ATP
1937 AD	Description of the Krebs cycle
1941 AD	Identification of ATP as primary energy transfer molecule
1945 AD	Identification of acetyl coenzyme A
1945–1951 AD	Localization of oxidative phosphorylation to the mitochondria

the blood.[3,4] Although some investigators have argued that this understanding was complete, others have shown that the Chinese understanding was limited but on par with their Western contemporaries.[4] There is also evidence that the ancient Indian cultures were beginning to investigate and conceptualize circulation at this time (approximately 600 BC).[3,5] All these early investigators described aspects of circulation, but no overarching understanding emerged during this time. Several theories from this early age of discovery led to centuries of stagnation.

The Greeks

The work of the ancient Greeks highlights the erratic nature of the early efforts to categorize the anatomy and physiology of the circulatory system. In a burst of effort from 400 to 200 BC, Greek scientists and philosophers (often one and the same) set forth several observations and theories regarding the circulatory system. Hippocrates made suggestions of the "circulatory" nature of the cardiovascular system[2] and that the heart was a muscle.[1] Aristotle identified the heart as the seat of physiologic mechanisms.[6] Praxagoras differentiated veins and arteries.[6] Erasistratus espoused that the heart was the source of both veins and arteries[6] and identified the tricuspid valve and the chordae tendineae.[1] Yet, although there was validity in these observations, they were surrounded by theories that provided as many false steps as advances. Hippocratic medicine focused on the concept of the 4 humors, with blood only a component of the balance and blending of forces necessary for health and life[2] and the circulation centering on the warming and cooling of the blood by the heart and lungs.[3]

Empedocles identified the liver as the source of the blood, leading to the organ identified as a major component of the circulatory system in early theories.[1] Erasistratus believed that there were 2 circulations, with the liver and the heart acting as sources of flow of the blood.[1] He also espoused, as did several other theorists of the day, that the arteries carried air, or the "spirit of life," from the lungs to the body as the second portion of the circulation.[1,6,7] Thus, although the early Greek intellectuals set the stage for the description of the basic components of the circulatory system, and thus the basis of tissue perfusion, their conceptualization of the flow through the system was flawed. These concepts of dual circulation, delivery of air to the tissues, and the balance of humors were the extent of understanding of the circulatory system for the next approximately 400 years.

Galen of Pergamon

Galen of Pergamon, a physician and scientist of the second century, played a key role in further developing the understanding of the cardiovascular system. Although other systems of medical understanding continued to develop and be practiced around the world, modern Western medicine largely traces itself through this figure in Roman history. Galen built on the theories of the Greeks before him but used experimentation and observation to refine and systematize hippocratic medicine.[6] As an example, his experiments revealed that blood, not air, flowed through the arteries.[1,6,7] He was limited, however, by the technology and social norms of the day.[6] Although he dispelled the concept of direct delivery of air to the tissues, he could not perform systematic dissection nor examine tissue at the microscopic level. As a result, although Galen corrected some of the early misconceptions of the Greeks, he introduced a new series of problems to the understanding of the circulatory system and tissue perfusion.

In Galen's conceptualization, food was taken up from the intestines to the liver. Here the food was converted into blood, which then flowed to the heart. This flow was centrifugal in nature[1] and did not rely on pumping action from the organs (although he correctly identified the heart as having innate motion that was transmitted through the arteries, thus producing the sensation of the pulse).[1,6] The blood carried the vital spirit derived from the digestion of food.[6] Meanwhile, the lungs took in a vital force from the air.[6,7] The heart was the source of heat in the body and provided a mixing point for the two forces to combine and produce life. In Galen's understanding, again highlighting the lack of advanced anatomic study, tiny pores connected the right and left side of the heart and allowed this mixing to occur.[1,6,7] Whereas Erasistratus believed in two separate circulations in the body, Galen identified that the two were comingled, with the heart the mixing source. These galenic refinements corrected a few of the prior errors in the description of the circulation but produced a new set of issues.

Owing to the quirks of history, galenic medicine held sway through the Western world for more than 1000 years. Several societal and historical influences prevented any further advancement in the Western understanding of tissue perfusion. Galen's work was endorsed by the church and gained an unassailable status in Christian culture.[6] When combined with prohibitions on dissection and the overall inability to engage in intellectual works during the Dark Ages, advancement of the understanding of perfusion stagnated in the Western world.

The Arabic World

The advancement of understanding, however, did not stop everywhere during this time. As Europe entered into a period of intellectual stagnation, the science of the Arabic world began to blossom and thrive. Although contributions to math and architecture are widely recognized, advancements in medicine abounded as well. The

Arabic world had been heavily influenced by the knowledge of the early Greeks and continued to build on those early theories. In the ninth century, Abu Bakr Mohammad Zakariya Razi wrote in his book, *Tebb-e Mansouri*, about the anatomy of the heart and great vessels, with details that far exceeded those found in Western writing for centuries.[3] During the tenth century, Avicenna (Ibn Sina) produced one of the most comprehensive treatises on medicine perhaps ever written by one author, in his *Canon of Medicine* (**Fig. 1**). This work remained one of the major medical texts of the medieval era.[8] Avicenna reinforced and codified earlier galenic and hippocratic medicine, while giving greater emphasis to the position and function of the heart. He also placed great importance on the connection between the pulse and breathing patterns and diseases of the heart and emphasized the observation of the vital signs in understanding the wellness of the patient.[9] This emphasis remained the basis for understanding and monitoring tissue perfusion for the next several centuries.

Although Avicenna was recognized as a major contributor to the study of medicine for centuries to come, his contributions were not the only important contributions from the Arabic world during this time. The first challenges to the galenic principles began to appear in the Middle East during the thirteenth century. Ibn al-Nafis became a prominent physician and scientist in Egypt during this period. He built on the work of Avicenna but refused to accept his predecessors' works as authoritative and challenged the anatomic assumptions of Galen[7,10] and others. In doing so, he preceded the challenges of Renaissance researchers by several hundred years.[8] Ibn al-Nafis' writings directly contradict the earlier galenic theory that the right and left heart must be connected by microscopic pores through the septum.[7,8] Instead, al-Nafis argued that the blood must flow from the right ventricle through small connections in the lungs to the left ventricle.[8] He also identified that the heart has its own vascular supply as part of

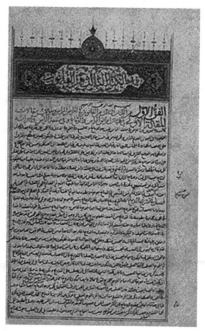

Fig. 1. The front page of a manuscript by Avicenna. (*From* Ibn Sina Gallery. Available at: http://www.muslimphilosophy.com/sina/gal/IS-gal-14.htm. Accessed April 23, 2014.)

this circulation.[7] These writings in the *Commentary on the Anatomy in Avicenna's Canon* are now recognized as the first written description of the pulmonary and myocardial circulation.[6] This major contribution was, unfortunately, not well disseminated due to language barriers and tensions between Europe and the Arabic world and did not reach the West in translation from Arabic to Latin until the 1500s.[6,8] By that point, Western scientists were beginning to mount their own challenges as the Dark Ages ended and the science of perfusion pushed forward.

The Renaissance

Considerable debate exists as to the influence that the Arabic writings played on the advancement of the science of perfusion in the Western world during the Renaissance period.[3,6,10] Aird[6] points out that around the time of al-Nafis' work, dissection of animals was undertaken in a systematic way in Salerno, Italy. This was followed more than a century later with the dissection of humans in Bologna, Italy. These anatomic studies were undertaken not as scientific endeavors but to demonstrate and teach galenic principles.[6] It was not until the mid-1500s that the first true challenges to the anatomy of Galen were made in the Western world. During this period, an explosion of investigators altered the understanding of the anatomy of the circulatory system and the flow through it. Andreas Vesalius, Miguel Servetus, and Realdo Colombo are all credited with duplicating the confirmation of the lack of pores between the right and left heart, as originally posited by al-Nafis.[6,8,10] Evidence rapidly accumulated confirming that blood flowed through a circuit from the right heart to the left through the lungs and not via an intracardiac pathway. Additional details of the cardiopulmonary anatomy, including the presence of coronary valves by da Vinci,[1] competence of the coronary valves by Colombo,[6] identification of the vena cava as not originating in the liver but rather the heart by Cesalpinus,[1] and the presence of venous valves by Canano and Estienne[1] and their competence by Fabricius,[6] further brought clarity to the understanding of the gross anatomy of the circulatory system. With the tenets of Galen's anatomy now firmly under fire, the first major leap in the understanding of circulation and perfusion was possible for the first time in a millennium in the West.

William Harvey

Modern Western medicine traces its understanding of the circulation of blood and perfusion of the tissues to the work of William Harvey in his 1628 *Exercitatio Anatomica de Motu Cordis et Sanguinis in Animalibus*. Harvey's studies firmly established the unidirectional flow of blood through the heart, lungs, and blood vessels and finally replaced Galen's theory.[10] He removed any possibility of intracardiac connections between the sides of the heart. Although he was not able to directly view them, Harvey surmised that there must be microscopic connections in the lungs that linked the blood flow on the right and left sides of the heart.[6] He demonstrated that blood passes to the tissues by the arteries and returns via the veins, surmising that there must be microscopic connections between the two in the tissues themselves.[6] He removed the liver from the system as a pump, as had been espoused by many early authors.[10] Although some pieces were still missing in description, his findings left the heart as the only driver of flow in the circulatory system and confirmed a single continuous circulatory flow for the first time.

Harvey's contribution to advancing understanding extended beyond the macroscopic anatomy of the circulatory system. Although the study of perfusion had taken millennia to outline the basic path of blood flow from the heart through the body and back again, another key piece prevented understanding of the purpose of this flow. Until the time of Harvey, blood was viewed as a nutrient force that was assembled from the building blocks taken from food in the intestines. Blood was believed to be produced in the liver and consumed by the tissues. Harvey calculated that the volume of blood passing through the heart, in a now unidirectional flow, in a short period of time was greater than the entire volume of blood in the body. These calculations also proved that the volume of blood needed to meet this flow could not possibly come from the nutrition ingested in a day.[6,10] Thus, the blood was no longer consumed during the circulation but ran the course continuously through the circuit. The Greek humoral theory was finally being called into question.

Harvey also used his experiments and new understanding of the circulatory anatomy to call into question one other major component of galenic medicine. The arteries were believed to carry air directly from the lungs to the tissue. In addition, "vapors" were believed to move from the organs to the lungs by the pulmonary veins and be expelled. Harvey found only blood in the arteries and concluded that air was not directly carried to the tissues as a "vital force."[6] Likewise, the vapors could not move backward through the system. He took this a step further and decided that the heart was not the place of mixing of blood and air but rather that the lungs were.[10] No longer were vital forces flowing back and forth to the heart and lungs through the arteries but rather were carried through the continuous flow within the arteries and veins.

Microscopic Anatomy

Although Harvey's theory addressed the macroscopic circulation needed to understand perfusion, his theory implied microscopic connections that had yet to be confirmed. The reliance on unseen microscopic anatomy left his theory to be questioned for the next several decades. To an extent, the concept of the macroscopic anatomy had been limited by the inability of investigators to look for and disprove the pores that Galen had theorized were present in the septum. The invention of the microscope opened new avenues of refinement for Renaissance investigators.[11] The understanding of circulation and perfusion now turned to the microscopic anatomy. Marcello Malpighi, a contemporary of Harvey, made 3 critical discoveries using early microscopes that removed many of the roadblocks to the acceptance of Harvey's theory (**Fig. 2**). His research confirmed the presence of the elusive pulmonary capillaries and provided the first description of the connection between the arterial and venous beds[11] that was needed to erase the doubts of Harvey's theory. These capillary beds brought the flow of blood into close proximity to the second of his monumental discoveries, the alveolus (**Fig. 3**). His description of the alveolus changed the understanding of the anatomy and physiology of the lung in dramatic fashion.[11] The anatomy he described demonstrated the separation of the blood from the air.[12] This finished the concept that the air was carried directly to the tissues by the arteries. Finally, Malpighi described the presence of individual red cells in the blood, thus introducing the basic nature of the blood. Although other researchers further refined and enhanced Harvey's theory, the microscopic anatomy needed to complete Harvey's anatomic theory was completed within a century of his death. These anatomic discoveries documented the development of various circulatory models, leading to the current anatomic circulatory model (**Fig. 4**).

PHYSIOLOGY AND BIOCHEMISTRY ERA

The development of modern concepts of perfusion now turns away from the earlier struggles to define the anatomy of the circulatory system and toward the sciences of physiology and early biochemistry. The basic processes of perfusion were

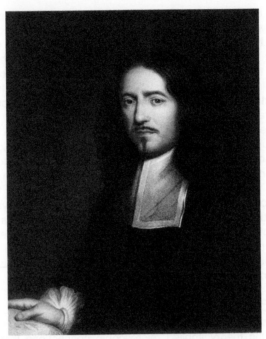

Fig. 2. Marcello Malpighi (1628–1694). (*From* West JB. Marcello Malpighi and the discovery of the pulmonary capillaries and alveoli. Am J Physiol Lung Cell Mol Physiol 2013;304:L383–90.)

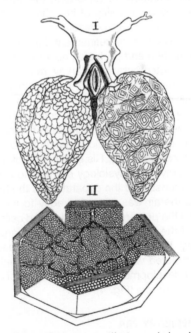

Fig. 3. Malpighi's drawing of the pulmonary capillaries and alveoli. (I) Lungs with the alveoli on the left and the capillaries on the right. (II) Pulmonary capillaries in a diagram of an alveolus that has been opened up. (*From* Malpighi M. De pulmonibus. London: Philosophic Transactions of the Royal Society; 1661.)

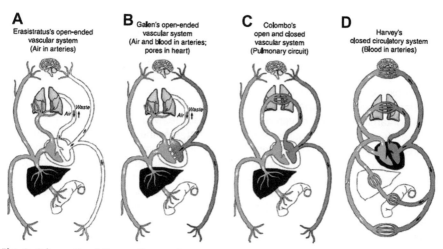

A Erasistratus's open-ended vascular system (Air in arteries)

B Galen's open-ended vascular system (Air and blood in arteries; pores in heart)

C Colombo's open and closed vascular system (Pulmonary circuit)

D Harvey's closed circulatory system (Blood in arteries)

Fig. 4. Schematic of the cardiovascular system over time. (*A*) According to Erasistratus, arteries and veins are separate. Veins contain blood (*blue color*), whereas arteries contain air (*white color*). Food is taken up in the intestines by the portal veins, delivered to the liver (*black color*), transformed into blood, and then transported to the vena cava by way of the hepatic vein. From the vena cava, venous blood is delivered to all parts of the body. Some of the blood is diverted to the right ventricle (*blue colored chamber in the heart*), from where it enters the pulmonary artery to nourish the lungs. Air is taken up in the lungs by the pulmonary veins, transferred to the left ventricle and distributed to the tissues via the arteries. Fuliginous vapors (waste) ate excreted by retrograde flow through the mitral valve and pulmonary vein. (*B*) Galen demonstrated that arteries normally contain blood (*red color*), not air. Arterial blood is derived from the passage of venous blood through invisible pores in the interventricular septum (shown as interrupted septal wall). (*C*) Colombo described the pulmonary circuit, in which venous blood in the right ventricle passes through the lungs into the left ventricle and arteries. Colombo maintained, however, the Ancient Greek view that blood flow in veins is centrifugal (away from the liver and toward all tissues), with only a small amount entering the right heart. Thus, Colombo's system is a hybrid between closed (pulmonary) and open (systemic). (*D*) Harvey discovered that blood circulates not only in the lung but also around the whole body. An important clue was the presence of valves in the veins (2 of them are shown in *white*). The liver is no longer the source of veins. Rather, the system is driven by the mechanics of the heart (now shown in *black*). Transfer of blood from arteries to veins in the lung and periphery may occur through direct connections or anastomoses (as shown) or through porosities in the flesh (the latter mechanism favored by Harvey). (*From* Aird WC. Discovery of the cardiovascular system: from Galen to William Harvey. J Thromb Haemost 2011;9(Suppl 1):120; with permission.)

represented in Galen's vision of the circulatory system in ancient times[6] in more mystical than scientific frames. The mystical nature of the process remained part of later systems of understanding because the basic science needed to explain the conversion of food and breath to life and energy did not yet exist. Starting in the late eighteenth century, the early days of the Industrial Revolution saw the development of several chemical breakthroughs in support of the growing industrial complex. These breakthroughs were rapidly applied to the study of perfusion.

Oxygen and Hemoglobin

The early chemical discovery most relevant to the history of perfusion is that of oxygen, which was made by two competing researchers: Joseph Priestley and

Antoine Lavoisier. Joseph Priestley isolated oxygen while experimenting with red mercuric oxide in 1774.[13,14] This produced a clear odorless gas that triggered enhanced burning in embers and supported the life of a mouse for longer than normal air alone.[14] Unfortunately, Priestley misinterpreted his development, believing that he had driven off a theoretic contaminant called phlogiston.[13] Reportedly, Carl Wilhelm Scheele had isolated oxygen even earlier but had failed to release his findings.[14] Priestley's rival Lavoisier repeated the experiment and recognized that a gas was produced rather than a contaminant being driven off. He and his wife, Marie-Anne, experimented on this new element. In the course of their experiments, the Lavoisiers demonstrated the existence of oxygen. They confirmed that oxygen was a necessary component of combustion. This provided insight to the process of combustion and other energy-releasing chemical reactions. Later Lavoisier turned his attention to the "vital" processes found in physiology. In 1783, Lavoisier, in association with Pierre-Simon Laplace, designed and used an ice calorimeter with guinea pigs to determine that "*la respiration est donc une combustion, à la vérité fort lente*" ("respiratory gas exchange is a combustion, a slow one to be precise").[15] This discovery was the first recognition of the aerobic biochemical processes of life and identified the central role of oxygen in metabolism.

Characterizations of the molecule hemoglobin started approximately a century after the discovery of oxygen with the observations of Hünefeld that the blood of earthworms formed crystals when dried in 1840. Hünefeld and other researchers further identified the molecule in the blood of other species.[16] George Stokes is credited for discovering the respiratory function of hemoglobin.[16] With the characterization of hemoglobin as a molecule involved in carrying oxygen to the tissues and the presence of hemoglobin in blood cells, there was now an explanation for the delivery of oxygen on red cells to the tissues and the transport of carbon dioxide, released as part of the combustion of respiration, to the lungs. The basic groundwork on the perfusion of tissues was established by the end of the nineteenth century.

With the recognition that blood, including hemoglobin, was necessary for oxygen delivery and carbon dioxide removal, investigators sought new methods for studying organ blood flow. Oskar Langendorf developed the isolated heart preparation in 1895, which allowed a beating heart to be examined in vitro while maintaining a heartbeat while outside the body.[17] This technique continues to be used for the examination of cardiac function and pharmacologic actions of medications on cardiac muscle. This research preparation also provided a way to study isolated perfused organs and to examine their response to various perfusion strategies. This was a primary technique for cardiac examination in vitro until in vivo examination via echocardiography was described by Edler and Hertz in 1953.[18]

Cellular Metabolism

Since the late 1800s and early 1900s, much of the focus on perfusion has shifted from an anatomic and gross physiologic approach to a focus on understanding the biochemistry associated with tissue metabolism. The biochemical pathways that produce and transform energy are numerous and complex. Considering cellular respiration from a historical perspective, numerous, perhaps thousands, of investigators have played a role in developing this knowledge. Several figures have played prominent roles in the discovery of these biochemical pathways.

ATP is probably one of the most important molecules in the biochemistry of human perfusion and metabolism. ATP was originally discovered in 1899 by Karl Lohmann (**Fig. 5**).[19] The significance of the ATP molecule was not completely understood until 1941 when Albert Lippman suggested that ATP may be the primary molecule to

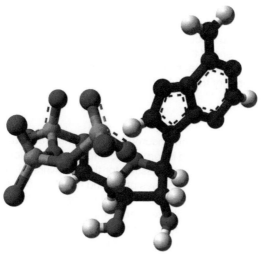

Fig. 5. 3-D reconstruction of structure of ATP.

transfer energy within the body. These discoveries drove the modern understanding of physiologic ATP production and its utilization for the "work" of cellular processes.

In 1937, Hans Krebs first described the citric acid cycle (now more commonly known as the Krebs cycle), which is a series of chemical reactions that generate a portion of biochemical energy through the oxidation of fatty acids, amino acids, and carbohydrates.[20] Elements of this cycle had been previously identified by other well-known biochemists, but Krebs ultimately put the pieces together to identify the entire biochemical cycle.

Lippman went on to discover the role of acetyl coenzyme A in 1945, which provides the chemical link for carbohydrates, fatty acids, and amino acids to enter into the Krebs cycle.[21] This provided the biochemical route for food substrates to be oxidized for biochemical energy within a cell. In combination with Krebs' discovery, this laid the foundation for the modern understanding of cell metabolism. Together, Krebs and Lippman were awarded the Nobel Prize in Physiology or Medicine in 1953.[21]

During that same time frame of the 1940's and 50's, a group of researchers were working to discover the biochemical links between the Krebs cycle and ATP production.[22] From 1945 to 1951, several important discoveries were made by Albert Lehninger and his colleagues. Lehninger and Eugene Kennedy went on to discover that most of the oxidative phosphorylation of substrates occurred in the mitochondria of cells.[22] Although previous work suggested that the mitochondria played an important role in energy production, Lehninger and Kennedy confirmed the mitochondria as the primary cell structure in which energy is produced. As a continued expansion of this work, Lehninger along with Morris Friedkin went on to discover the electron transport chain and identify nicotinamide adenine dinucleotide as one of the biochemical links between the Krebs cycle and the electron transport chain.[23]

When looking at these biochemical processes, it is important to understand the link to the concept of perfusion. Carbon dioxide production, and ultimately its removal as a waste product from the body, is central to perfusion. Carbon dioxide is produced during the formation of acetyl coenzyme A and during the Krebs cycle. Once carbon dioxide is released, it forms carbonic acid, which can reduce body fluid pH and interfere with enzyme-based intracellular biochemical processes when not removed. This is the fundamental cause of death from uncompensated hypercarbic respiratory failure. Oxygen also plays a role within these biochemical processes as the final electron acceptor at the end of the electron transport chain. If oxygen is not present to accept this final electron at the end of the electron transport chain, the movement of electrons is halted and the process is unable to produce ATP. This is the fundamental cause of death occurring secondary to cellular hypoxia.

SUMMARY

The modern concept of perfusion encompasses a variety of anatomic, physiologic, and biochemical ideas. These are incorporated into a model of how the body delivers fuel substrates and oxygen to target tissues for their conversion into energy that the body uses for the biochemical processes of life and how the body removes the waste byproducts that occur during these biochemical processes. This modern concept of perfusion has largely grown out of discoveries that have taken centuries of scientific inquiry. The concept of tissue perfusion continues to evolve and develop. This article discussed a few of the important people and events that helped to develop the modern concept of perfusion. Although the basic groundwork of tissue perfusion was completed by the middle of the twentieth century, there continue to be discoveries and refinements of understanding. As the means of exploring the intracellular milieu improve, additional links become apparent. These new discoveries are also opening the door to new ways to bring theoretic knowledge to bedside monitoring and care.

REFERENCES

1. Garrison F. An outline of the history of the circulatory system. Bull N Y Acad Med 1931;7(10):781–806.
2. Cheng TO. Hippocrates, cardiology, Confucius and the Yellow Emperor. Int J Cardiol 2001;81:219–33.
3. Azizi MH, Nayernouri T, Azizi F. A brief history of the discovery of the circulation of blood in the human body. Arch Iran Med 2008;11(3):345–50.
4. Jing-Bao N. Refutation of the claim that the ancient Chinese described the circulation of blood: a critique of scientism in the historiography of Chinese medicine [Internet]. N Z J Asian Stud 2001;3(2):119–35. Available at: http://www.nzasia.org.nz/downloads/NZJAS-Dec01/Jingbao.pdf.
5. Dwivedi G, Dwivedi S. Sushruta – the clinician – teacher par excellence. Indian J Chest Dis Allied Sci 2007;49:243–4.
6. Aird WC. Discovery of the cardiovascular system: from Galen to William Harvey. J Thromb Haemost 2011;9(Suppl 1):118–29.
7. Haddad SI, Khairallah AA. A forgotten chapter in the history of the circulation of the blood. Ann Surg 1936;104:1–8.
8. West JB. Ibn al-Nafis, the pulmonary circulation and the Islamic Golden Age. J Appl Physiol (1985) 2008;105:1877–80.
9. Turgut O, Manhduz S, Tandogan I. Avicenna: messages from a great pioneer of ancient medicine for modern cardiology. Int J Cardiol 2010;145(2):222.
10. Martins e Silva J. Da descoberta da Circulação Sanguínea aos Primeiros Factos Hemorreológicos (1ª Parte). [From the discovery of the circulation of the blood to the first steps in hemorheology: part 1]. Rev Port Cardiol 2009;28(11):1245–68 [in Portuguese].
11. West JB. Marcello Malpighi and the discovery of the pulmonary capillaries and alveoli. Am J Physiol Lung Cell Mol Physiol 2013;304:L383–90.

12. Martins e Silva J. Da descoberta da Circulação Sanguínea aos Primeiros Factos Hemorreológicos (2ª Parte). [From the discovery of the circulation of the blood to the first steps in hemorheology: part 2]. Rev Port Cardiol 2009;28(12): 1405–40 [in Portuguese].
13. Fara P. Joseph Priestley: doctor phlogiston or reverend oxygen? Endeavor 2010; 34(3):84–6.
14. West JB. The collaboration of Antoine and Marie-Anne Lavoisier and the first measurements of human oxygen consumption. Am J Physiol Lung Cell Mol Physiol 2013;305(11):L775–85.
15. Buchholz AC, Schoeller DA. Is a calorie a calorie? Am J Clin Nutr 2004;79(5): 899S–906S.
16. Ferry RM. Studies in the chemistry of hemoglobin 1: the preparation of hemoglobin. J Biol Chem 1923;57:819–28.
17. Broadley KJ. The Langendorff heart preparation—Reappraisal of its role as a research and teaching model for coronary vasoactive drugs. J Pharmacol Methods 1979;2(2):143–56.
18. Singh S, Goyal A. The origin of echocardiography: a tribute to Inge Edler. Tex Heart Inst J 2007;34(4):431–8.
19. Langen P, Hucho F. Karl Lohmann and the discovery of ATP. Angew Chem Int Ed Engl 2008;47(10):1824–7.
20. Kornberg H. Krebs and his trinity of cycles. Nat Rev Mol Cell Biol 2000;1(3): 225–8.
21. Buchanan JM. Biochemistry during the life and times of Hans Krebs and Fritz Lipmann. J Biol Chem 2002;277(37):33531–6.
22. Daniel Lane M, Talalay P. Albert Lester Lehninger. J Membr Biol 1986;91(3): 193–7.
23. Kresge N, Simoni RD, Hill RL. The ATP requirement for fatty acid oxidation: the early work of Albert L. Lehninger. J Biol Chem 2005;280(14):e11.

Microcirculatory Oxygen Transport and Utilization

Shannan K. Hamlin, PhD, RN, ACNP-BC, AGACNP-BC, CCRN[a,*],
C. Lee Parmley, MD, JD, MMHC[b,c], Sandra K. Hanneman, PhD, RN[d]

KEYWORDS

- Microcirculation • Oxygen transport • Oxygen utilization • Oxygen extraction
- Capillary • Blood flow • Hemodynamics

KEY POINTS

- The microcirculation is a complex system designed to ensure that oxygen delivery meets or exceeds cellular oxygen demand.
- The cardiovascular system (macrocirculation) circulates blood throughout the body but the microcirculation, with its 10 billion capillaries, is responsible for modifying tissue perfusion and adapting it to metabolic demand.
- Hemodynamic assessment and monitoring of the critically ill patient is typically focused on global measures of oxygen transport and utilization, which do not evaluate the status of the microcirculation.
- Despite achievement and maintenance of global hemodynamic and oxygenation goals, patients may develop microcirculatory dysfunction with associated organ failure.
- A thorough understanding of the microcirculatory system under physiologic conditions will assist the clinician in early recognition of microcirculatory dysfunction in impending and actual disease states.

INTRODUCTION

Claude Bernard (1813–1878), a nineteenth-century French physiologist, was the first to publish a recognition that all higher-level organisms constantly strive to maintain internal homeostasis by actively controlling such variables as temperature, oxygen concentration, composition of ions, osmolality, and pH.[1] As strictly aerobic living

Funding Sources: None.
Conflict of Interest: None.
[a] Nursing Research and Evidence-Based Practice, Houston Methodist Hospital, MGJ 11-017, Houston, TX 77030, USA; [b] Vanderbilt University Hospital, 1211 21st Avenue South, S3408 MCN, Nashville, TN 37212, USA; [c] Department of Anesthesiology, Division of Critical Care, Vanderbilt University School of Medicine, 1211 21st Avenue South, S3408 MCN, Nashville, TN 37212, USA; [d] University of Texas Health Science Center at Houston School of Nursing, Center for Nursing Research, Room #594, 6901 Bertner Avenue, Houston, TX 77030, USA
* Corresponding author.
E-mail address: SHamlin@HoustonMethodist.org

organisms, human beings depend on oxygen for survival. As such, aerobic metabolism and organ function rely on the delivery and distribution of adequate amounts of oxygen. In the struggle against biological death from any cause, the battle is won or lost based on the restoration of adequate oxygen delivery (Do_2) and oxygen consumption (Vo_2).[2] To accomplish this goal, a complex oxygen transport network involving the lungs, heart, macrovasculature, and microvasculature work in concert to receive oxygen from the environment and transport it to the tissues for utilization. Blood flow through the large blood vessels and microvasculature is referred to macrocirculation and microcirculation, respectively.

The microcirculation is a complex and integrated system that ensures oxygen delivery meets or exceeds cellular oxygen demand. The cardiovascular system, with its large arteries and veins, circulates blood throughout the body, but it is the microcirculation that regulates blood flow and distribution of red blood cells (RBCs) throughout individual organs.[3] Indeed, the microcirculation, with its 10 billion capillaries, is responsible for adjusting tissue perfusion to adapt to varying metabolic demands.[4] Despite this critical role, until recently the microcirculation has been neglected in practice. Hemodynamic assessment of the critically ill patient focuses on such global measures of oxygen transport and utilization such as cardiac output, arterial blood pressure, Do_2, and Vo_2, none of which assesses the status of the microcirculation. Microcirculatory failure can occur despite the achievement and maintenance of normal, or even supranormal, systemic hemodynamic and oxygenation goals. A thorough understanding of the microcirculatory system under physiologic conditions is prerequisite to understanding the microcirculation in disease states. This article reviews the microcirculatory system, focusing on the anatomy and physiology of oxygen transport and utilization.

ANATOMY AND PHYSIOLOGY OF CIRCULATION

Broadly stated, the function of the heart and larger blood vessels is to pump and carry blood to and from the body's organs and tissues; the macrocirculation delivers blood to and receives blood from the microcirculation. The microcirculation, composed of specific vessels to be discussed subsequently, distributes the blood to regions of the body where it is needed and away from regions where it is not, then collects and returns it to the macrocirculation.[5]

Oxygenated blood leaving the pulmonary capillary system enters the left heart to be ejected to the systemic circulation. After leaving the heart, blood travels from the aorta to arteries that become progressively smaller until reaching the arterioles, then the capillaries, venules, and veins, each distinguished from each other by physical dimensions, characteristic morphology, and specific function.[1] Before blood travels back to the right heart, deoxygenated and ready to repeat the process, its real business has occurred during its course through the microcirculation. The microcirculation consists of the arterioles, capillaries, and venules. These vessels deliver and distribute oxygen, nutrients (eg, glucose and fatty acids), and inflammatory and coagulation factors to the tissues, and remove waste products of metabolism (eg, carbon dioxide and heat) (**Fig. 1**).[3,6]

Arterioles

The first vessels of the microcirculation are arterioles, which receive blood from arteries of the macrocirculation. Arterioles are referred to as resistance vessels because of their ability to constrict and dilate so as to regulate blood flow to individual organs. Arterioles have an endothelial lining with a thick smooth muscle layer and a thin

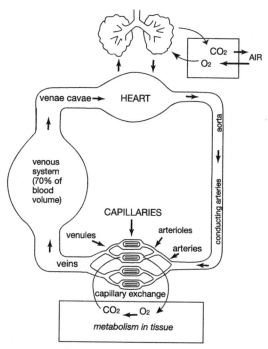

Fig. 1. Role of the macrovascular and microvascular systems in oxygen transport. Newly oxygenated blood leaves the pulmonary circulation and enters the systemic circulation. The heart pumps oxygenated blood through the aorta to the arteries, then arterioles, before entering the capillaries where oxygen (O_2) and nutrients enter the tissues by diffusion for use in metabolism. Carbon dioxide (CO_2) and other waste products leave the tissues and enter the capillaries for removal first via venules, then veins. The veins act as a storage system, holding up to 70% of the total blood volume. (*From* Opie LH. Introductory cardiovascular concepts. The heart physiology, from cell to circulation. 3rd edition. Philadelphia: Lippincott-Raven; 1998. p. 8; with permission.)

adventitial layer; their internal diameter is approximately 30 μm with a wall thickness of 20 μm.[7] As the source of peripheral or systemic vascular resistance (SVR), the arterioles provide the major source of resistance the cardiac ventricles must overcome to pump blood into the circulation.[6] As arterioles dilate, SVR decreases and more blood enters the capillaries they supply; conversely, as the arterioles constrict, less blood enters the capillaries.[6] The significance of vessel diameter or radius (r = d/2) is apparent in Poiseuille's law, which relates velocity of blood flow within a vessel to the vessel's radius to the fourth power. The complex balance of constriction and dilation of arterioles to assure blood is directed to capillary beds in the location and quantity appropriate to meet the body's needs is regulated through neuronal and humeral means. These principles are discussed in more detail later.

Capillaries

Capillaries receive blood delivered by arterioles. Capillaries are exchange vessels, where oxygenated blood becomes deoxygenated as oxygen chemically dissociates from the hemoglobin (Hgb) molecule, to then diffuse out of the RBCs through the plasma to the capillary wall.[6,8] Oxygen diffuses through the capillary wall to reach the tissue mitochondria, where energy is produced by oxidative phosphorylation.[8]

This biochemical process is a basic reaction whereby oxygen is used to produce energy by[8]:

$$3 \text{ ADP} + 3 \text{ Pi} + 1/2 \text{ O}_2 + \text{NADH} + \text{H}^+ \rightarrow 3 \text{ ATP} + \text{NAD}^+ + \text{H}_2\text{O}$$

where ADP and ATP are adenosine diphosphate and triphosphate, respectively; Pi is inorganic phosphate; NADH and NAD^+ are reduced and oxidized forms of nicotinamide adenine dinucleotide, respectively; H^+ is a hydrogen ion; and H_2O is water.[8]

Capillaries are the smallest microvascular vessels, with an internal diameter of approximately 5 μm and a single-layer wall thickness of 1 μm.[9] Capillaries contain no smooth muscle, and therefore lack the ability to actively change their diameter. The capillary is the primary site of oxygen exchange within the tissue. The distribution of capillaries, or capillary density, varies within and among tissues according to the oxygen requirements for the metabolic needs of specific tissues and organs.[7] In more metabolically active tissues, such as cardiac and skeletal muscles, the capillary density is high in comparison with less active tissues such as subcutaneous tissue.[7]

A large range of flow resistance per unit length exists among capillaries, which results in heterogeneous blood flow within various capillary beds.[10] Capillary network geometry not only affects blood-flow distribution but also predicts in which capillary segments flow will cease when arterial perfusion pressure is reduced.[10] Using a rat model, Lindbom and Arfors[11] showed a gradual decrease in the number of perfused capillaries, despite a concomitant increase in terminal arteriolar diameters, as perfusion pressure was gradually decreased. Even with constant driving pressure (ie, arteriolar pressure), small capillary diameter around 5 μm impedes the flow of RBCs with a diameter around 8 μm.[10] That diameter, of course, is of the circular aspect of the discoid RBC; fortunately normal RBCs are flexible and deform to travel in single file through smaller capillary vessels, an effect that maximizes the RBC's surface area for optimal gas exchange at the capillary/tissue level.[3]

Capillary Density

Tissue perfusion is ultimately determined by blood flow and capillary density, which are associated with convective and diffusive oxygen transport (see later discussion).[4] In healthy conditions, capillaries are recruited to increase blood flow or "derecruited" to limit flow to tissues according to oxygen requirement. This process results in blood being preferentially shunted to tissues with high oxygen requirement.[4] Capillary density can increase as an adaptive response to chronic hypoxia[12] and strenuous exercise training.[13] This response to training or chronic stress is a process that takes weeks to occur.[4] With acute tissue hypoxia, capillary recruitment can occur to a limited degree.[4] In situations of acute hypoxia or hemorrhage, capillary density has been observed to increase up to 10%.[14]

Increased capillary density by recruitment increases the number of functional capillaries, the result of which is more oxygen available for the tissues. The effect of increased total oxygen reaching the tissue is an increase in tissue oxygen tension (Po_2), which reduces the critical oxygen diffusion distance, that is, the distance oxygen must diffuse from the capillary to reach the mitochondria where it will be utilized. The Po_2 gradient from the capillary to the tissue to the mitochondria is responsible for diffusive oxygen transport. With an increase in functional capillaries, more oxygen is received into the capillaries, and the Po_2 gradient increases. The Po_2 gradient facilitates oxygen dissociation from Hgb in tissues with high oxygen requirement, which will have a lower tissue Po_2. Consequently capillary density is greatest in tissues with high rates of oxygen consumption.[15]

The process of capillary recruitment in accordance with tissue demand provides local control of blood flow driven by backward communication, that is, from capillary to the arteriole, which is reflected in both upstream and downstream adaptation.[4] Several processes are thought to control arteriole and capillary adaptation through backward communication: (1) perivascular sympathetic nerves, which influence arteriolar tone upstream from capillaries[16]; (2) backward endothelial communication mediated by the endothelial cells themselves[4]; and (3) RBCs acting as intravascular oxygen sensors.[17]

Arteriolar Regulation

The microcirculation is regulated by the central nervous system and regional conditions in the direct vicinity of the specific vessel.[5] These regulatory influences are not homogeneous throughout all tissue beds. For example, in the splanchnic and integumentary tissues, neural regulation of blood flow predominates, whereas in the brain and heart, local influences predominate.[5]

Delivery of oxygen to tissues in a manner that meets changing metabolic needs involves a complex process of interplay between the pulmonary, cardiovascular, and microvascular systems, which globally alters blood flow according to inputs from the various neural, metabolic (regulation based on oxygen, carbon dioxide, lactate, and H^+), and myogenic (sensing strain and stress) controllers.[18] Regional controls, working parallel with global control systems, are in place to "sense" and respond when O_2 delivery in specific tissue beds within an individual organ is marginal.[19] To achieve the necessary degree of $\dot{D}o_2$ control for changing conditions (eg, increased oxygen demand, reduced oxygen delivery), the microvascular response must be highly integrated along the entire vascular bed.[15]

At rest, regulation of blood flow is largely controlled by the distal arterioles. As metabolic demands increase, larger arteries are recruited to regulate blood flow to the tissues.[20] This autoregulation of blood flow within specific tissue beds assures constant tissue metabolism or homeostasis by maintaining a nearly constant flow of oxygen-rich blood throughout a wide range of changing perfusion pressure and vascular resistance.[5]

Within an individual organ, arterioles control the vascular resistance and, therefore, the organ's total blood flow. In addition, however, they regulate the distribution of oxygen within the organ itself.[15] The density of functional capillaries must be high enough to ensure appropriate diffusion distances to meet tissue oxygen demand; however, it is the arteriolar regulation that distributes blood flow to where it is needed under variable conditions. In other words, it is not enough to simply supply an adequate amount of oxygen to an organ as a whole; the oxygen delivered must be distributed precisely to where it is needed according to tissue demand.[15]

Blood flow to capillary beds in the tissues tissue is actively controlled upstream through alterations in vascular tone, which affects the diameter of the arteriole.[3] Surrounded by smooth muscle, arterioles in response to local stimulation are able to constrict, restricting blood flow and increasing pressure, or dilate, decreasing pressure and increasing blood flow. In accordance with Poiseuille's law, capillary blood flow is inversely proportional to capillary length (L) and blood viscosity (η) and directly proportional to the driving pressure (ΔP) and the fourth power of the capillary radius (r), which corresponds to diameter ($r = d/2$)[4]:

Capillary flow $= \pi r^4\, \Delta P/8L\eta$

Considering that capillary length and viscosity cannot be actively manipulated, capillary flow can only be changed by local arteriolar vasodilation or vasoconstriction, resulting in an increased or decreased driving pressure to the capillary.[4] The significance of the effect of vascular resistance is apparent in the mathematical formula wherein flow is proportional to the fourth power of the vessel's radius. Although vessel diameter is the most influential factor,[21] resistance to flow is also influenced by blood viscosity and length of the vascular bed. Blood viscosity can alter resistance to blood flow; highly viscous blood (eg, in patients who are dehydrated or those with polycythemia) tends to "drag" in the vasculature and increase flow resistance,[21] whereas low-viscosity blood offers little resistance to flow.

Endothelium

The endothelial lining of the circulatory system is involved in numerous complex microcirculatory activities that include regulating the types and levels of homeostatic, vasoactive, and inflammatory agents in the blood, and modulating immune responses and vascular cell growth.[19,22] This highly specialized tissue also acts as a sensor, and therefore plays an active role in regulation of microvascular blood flow through the release of tissue hormones, such as the endothelial-derived relaxing autacoid prostacyclin (PGI_2), and the potent vasodilator nitric oxide, also known as endothelium-derived relaxing factor.[23,24] Stimulated by endothelial cell shear stress from blood flow, nitric oxide is synthesized from L-arginine and activates guanylyl cyclase in the vascular smooth muscle to increase the concentration of cyclic guanosine monophosphate (cGMP). The increase in cGMP results in relaxation of vascular smooth muscle by decreasing free Ca^{2+} in the cytosol.[7]

The endothelial cells that line the microvasculature play a crucial role in both conducting and integrating stimulatory signals via cell-to-cell communication[25] and by acting as signal transducers of local shear stress in response to changes in blood flow.[23] Because endothelial cells line the vascular lumen, these cells are the first cells exposed to environmental perturbations such as diminished oxygen.[22] For example, if an increase in shear stress (dilatory stimulus) is sensed in a specific region of a capillary bed, the endothelium will communicate this information to the arterioles supplying the capillary bed, causing the smaller arterioles to dilate and increase blood flow to the region. Endothelial cells lining larger arterioles further upstream also respond by dilating.

Red Blood Cell

The erythrocyte has an interesting role in the process of oxygen transport, largely as it functions to contain and integral components of the molecular processes such as Hgb and ATP. Within the RBC, oxygen binds to Hgb as it circulates from the lungs to the tissues, during which transit it changes from a high-oxygen-affinity structure to a low-oxygen-affinity structure. This transition in oxygen affinity promotes release, or dissociation, of oxygen from Hgb at the tissue level.[3] The characteristics of this oxygen affinity are reflected in the sigmoid shape of the oxyhemoglobin dissociation curve showing that the Hgb affinity for oxygen is affected by temperature, nitric oxide, pH, and carbon dioxide (**Fig. 2**).[3]

The RBC is more than an efficient carrier of Hgb, and thus oxygen, in the transport process. It also senses oxygen levels and releases ATP in response.[18] The RBC contains a large quantity of ATP, seemingly involved in maintenance of its characteristic deformability.[18] Bergfeld and Forrester[26] demonstrated that this reserve ATP in human RBCs can be released in response to hypoxia and hypercapnia, as occurs during vigorous exercise. The ATP released from RBCs binds with endothelial receptors, which alter vessel diameter.[18,27] ATP applied to arteriole lumens of hamster retractor muscles resulted in up to a 10% increase in vessel diameter upstream, and the

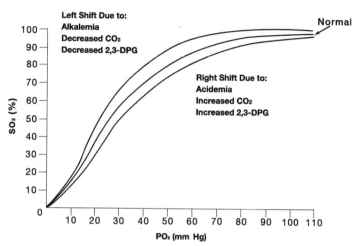

Fig. 2. Oxyhemoglobin dissociation curve showing the changing affinity of hemoglobin (Hgb) for oxygen related to the Po_2 of blood. Hgb binding with oxygen is increased (increased affinity) when the Po_2 is high, as at the pulmonary capillary. Conversely, oxygen readily dissociates from Hgb when the Po_2 is low, such as at the systemic capillaries. The oxyhemoglobin dissociation curve may be shifted right or left because of changes in the affinity of Hgb for oxygen. CO_2, carbon dioxide; DPG, diphosphoglycerate; Po_2, partial pressure of oxygen; So_2, oxygen saturation. (*Adapted from* Darovic GO, Zbilut JP. Pulmonary anatomy and physiology. In: Darovic GO, editor. Hemodynamic monitoring: invasive and noninvasive clinical application. 3rd edition. Philadelphia: W.B. Saunders Company; 2002. p. 35; with permission.)

increase in diameter was followed by an increase in tissue Po_2 of 3 mm Hg. This recognized effect of ATP on the microcirculation, considered in conjunction with the RBC's role in carrying ATP along with its responsive release of ATP, disclose the RBC's direct role in the regulation of vascular tone and microvascular flow.[18] Additional data suggest that RBCs may also be involved in regulating the distribution of microvascular perfusion in response to tissue hypoxia.[28]

Blood Flow

Whole blood is composed of cellular elements (eg, RBCs, leukocytes, platelets) suspended in liquid plasma. Viscosity is a property of blood that affects flow; it is determined by the hematocrit, which is essentially the ratio of the volume of cellular elements to the volume of whole blood.[29] Whole blood behaves as a non-Newtonian fluid when flowing through the circulatory system. High shear or frictional stresses along vessel walls finds the liquid or plasma component of blood there, where flow is slower than in the central aspect of the vessel where cellular elements tend to flow. As vessel diameter becomes smaller, the mean velocity of RBCs traveling through the vessel increases relative to plasma, as RBCs flow in single file in the central zone of the vessel and plasma flows peripherally where shear forces are greatest.

RBCs have an average diameter of 8 μm, but must traverse capillaries as small as 3 to 5 μm. Behaving as elastic bodies, RBCs respond to the pressure of small vessel diameter by changing their shape to allow movement through the vessel in single file.[30] This distinctive microvascular flow behavior maximizes the surface area available for gas exchange[1]; RBC deformability is the most important rheological factor affecting blood flow.[31] Worthy of consideration is the tendency for RBCs to clump together or aggregate. Aggregation increases flow resistance and viscosity, and is facilitated in low-shear conditions, especially those with increased levels of circulating fibrinogen, such as in sepsis.[3,32] Normally, however, high-velocity flow in the micro-vasculature discourages RBC aggregation.

FUNDAMENTALS OF OXYGEN TRANSPORT AND UTILIZATION

The microcirculation ensures that $\dot{D}o_2$ meets the metabolic oxygen demands of the tissues by actively and passively regulating the distribution of RBCs and plasma throughout individual organs.[3] Tissue oxygenation is adequate when demand is satisfied.[19] Four critical steps are involved in the process of oxygen transport: (1) bulk flow of oxygen from the environment to vascularized surfaces of the lungs; (2) diffusion of the oxygen from the pulmonary capillaries into the blood; (3) movement of oxygen in the arterialized blood to capillaries of organs and tissues of the body; and (4) diffusion of oxygen from the systemic capillaries through interstitial fluid, cytosol, and on to the mitochondria of each and every cell.[2] This 4-step process is separated into convective and diffusive aspects of oxygen transport.

Convective Oxygen Transport

The efficiency of oxygen transport, or the flow of oxygen from the lungs (high Po_2) to the tissues (low Po_2), involves convective and diffusive mechanisms.[3] Convective oxygen transport is the bulk transport of oxygen over large distances by the blood.[3] This mechanism of oxygen transport is calculated by considering the cardiac output (CO) and amount of oxygen in 100 mL of arterial blood (oxygen content [Cao_2]).[33] Arterial oxygen content is calculated by:

$$Cao_2 \text{ in vol\%} = Hgb \times Sao_2 \times 1.36$$

where Sao_2 is the arterial oxygen saturation and 1.36 is the number of cubic centimeters of oxygen a fully saturated gram of Hgb can carry. Physiologic arterial oxygen content is approximately 20 mL per 100 mL of whole blood (20 vol%); of this 20 mL of oxygen, 0.3 mL is dissolved in the plasma and 19.7 mL is bound to Hgb in the RBCs.[33] Oxygen transport can then be expressed as[2,33]:

$$O_2 \text{ transport} = CO \times Cao_2$$

Simply stated, convective oxygen transport determines the overall oxygen available for diffusion to the capillaries for intracellular utilization (**Fig. 3**).[33]

The volume and rate of arterial blood flow is determined by (1) the microvascular pressure gradient and (2) the resistance to flow.[21] Adequate blood flow will occur only if there is a sufficient pressure gradient or difference in pressure at both ends (pulmonary and systemic) of the circulation such that the magnitude of this gradient determines the driving force.

Diffusive Oxygen Transport

Diffusive oxygen transport is the process whereby oxygen moves from the microvasculature to the tissues and ultimately the mitochondria, where it is consumed. The direction of movement is determined exclusively by relative O_2 partial-pressure gradients; the movement of oxygen is from regions of higher Po_2 to areas of lower Po_2,[3] known as the capillary diffusion driving force.[34] Normal arteriole Po_2 is approximately 100 mm Hg, which is that entering the proximal end of the capillary beds. At the distal or venous end of the capillaries the Po_2 is about 20 mm Hg, which represents a diffusion gradient of 80 mm Hg across the capillary bed (arteriole Po_2 minus capillary

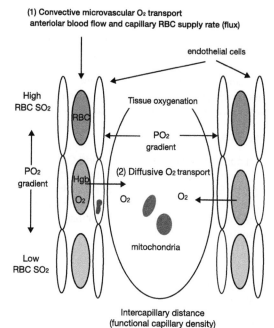

Fig. 3. Convective and diffusive oxygen transport in the microcirculation. Oxygen (O_2) is carried by the red blood cell (RBC; convective O_2 transport) from the lung microcirculation to the tissue microcirculation. As the RBC traverses the vascular bed, O_2 is offloaded to the tissue. Oxygen then diffuses from the capillary to the tissue mitochondria where it is consumed. Local oxygen tension (P_{O_2}) gradients are established (driving force of O_2 diffusion) along the capillary vessel as the RBC hemoglobin (Hgb) O_2 saturation (S_{O_2}) decreases. (*Adapted from* Bateman RM, Sharpe MD, Ellis CG. Bench-to-bedside review: microvascular dysfunction in sepsis-hemodynamics, oxygen transport, and nitric oxide. Crit Care 2003;7(5):362; with permission; and *Data from* Mohrman DE, Heller JJ. Overview of the cardiovascular system. Cardiovascular physiology. 5th edition. New York: Lange Medical Books/McGraw-Hill; 2003. p. 1–18.)

P_{O_2}) (see **Fig. 3**).[33] The diffusion gradient continues beyond the capillaries on to the mitochondria where oxygen is consumed, maintaining the low end of the P_{O_2} gradient. The P_{O_2} of mitochondria varies across a wide range among tissues, and in some may be in single-digit values.[35]

Independent of $\dot{D}_{O_2}$, oxygen diffusion is limited by the parameters of: (1) oxygen solubility (k); (2) oxygen diffusivity (D); (3) the P_{O_2} gradient (dP_{O_2}/dr); and (d) the critical oxygen diffusion distance, which is the maximum distance the mitochondria can be separated from an oxygen source without impaired function.[3] Oxygen diffusion is described mathematically using Fick's first law of diffusion (note that adding a negative sign in the expression [ie, $-kD$] changes the gradient's negative slope to a positive value for ease of interpretation[3]):

$$\text{Oxygen diffusion} = -kD \times dP_{O_2}/dr$$

Simply stated, adequate oxygen transport to the tissues depends on local microvascular oxygen delivery, the critical oxygen diffusion distance, and functional capillary density, as shown in **Fig. 3**.[3]

OXYGEN CONSUMPTION

$\dot{V}O_2$ is defined as the total amount of oxygen used by the body[36] per unit of time. Conceptually, $\dot{V}O_2$ accounts for the portion of oxygen delivered to the tissues ($\dot{D}O_2$) extracted during transit through the circuit from arterial to venous sides. Because the amount of oxygen delivered to the tissues ($\dot{D}O_2$) and the amount of oxygen returning to the heart (systemic mixed venous oxygen saturation [SvO_2]) are both measurable variables, the amount of oxygen consumed ($\dot{V}O_2$) can be estimated by the equation[2,33]:

$$\dot{V}O_2 = CO \times (CaO_2 \, [SaO_2] - CvO_2 \, [SvO_2])$$

where CaO_2 is oxygen content in the arterial blood and CvO_2 is oxygen content in the mixed venous blood. Because so little oxygen is unbound to Hgb, these parameters are measured clinically by SaO_2 and SvO_2, respectively. At times it is also clinically useful to consider the ratio of consumed oxygen to that delivered, the O_2 extraction ratio (O_2ER). O_2ER is defined as the fraction of $\dot{D}O_2$ that diffuses from the capillaries to the tissues, and is represented by the formula[2]:

$$O_2ER = \dot{V}O_2/\dot{D}O_2$$

Simplistically and practically this can be considered using the following application of monitored parameters:

$$O_2ER = (SaO_2 - SvO_2)/SaO_2$$

Ultimately, adequate tissue oxygenation therefore is a product of $\dot{D}O_2$ and O_2ER where oxygen demand is equal to $\dot{V}O_2$.[19] In other words:

$$O_2 \text{ demand} = \dot{V}O_2 = \dot{D}O_2 \times O_2ER$$

In the healthy adult, resting $\dot{D}O_2$ is approximately 1000 mL/min with about 25% (250 mL/min) consumed ($\dot{V}O_2$).[2] The O_2ER varies from tissue to tissue as blood flow to each organ is matched to metabolic requirements.[2,19] In times of increased O_2ER or decreased $\dot{D}O_2$, blood flow is redistributed among the organs, so that those organs capable of increasing O_2ER receive progressively smaller fractions of $\dot{D}O_2$ and those organs unable to increase O_2ER receive more blood flow.[19]

When $\dot{D}O_2$ is reduced by either decreased CaO_2 or arterial blood flow, compensatory mechanisms such as increased heart rate, respiratory rate, and myocardial contractility are activated to meet peripheral oxygen requirements.[19] Reductions in $\dot{V}O_2$ also stimulate these compensatory mechanisms to redistribute blood flow to vital organs.[19,37] The compensatory mechanisms help maintain $\dot{V}O_2$ by increasing O_2ER until a critical $\dot{D}O_2$ threshold is reached (approximately 4.5 mL/kg/min), which forces $\dot{V}O_2$ to become supply dependent. When $\dot{V}O_2$ is supply dependent, it will decrease with a progressive $\dot{D}O_2$ decline because O_2ER can no longer compensate for the deficit in $\dot{D}O_2$ (Fig. 4).[2,19] Decreased $\dot{V}O_2$ during critical oxygen-supply dependence represents true tissue dysoxia.[38]

In situations of increased oxygen demand, such as strenuous exercise, tissue $\dot{D}O_2$ is increased by both increased CO and increased oxygen extraction from hemoglobin.[39] The O_2ER can increase from a basal level of 0.25 to a maximum of 0.80. Although an O_2ER of 0.80 represents the point of maximum extraction, tissues transition from aerobic to anaerobic respiration at an O_2ER around 0.60.[39]

Maruyama and Fukuda[40] demonstrated in a rat model that there is a linear decline in $\dot{V}O_2$ accompanying a decline in $\dot{D}O_2$ when the $\dot{D}O_2$ values fall below 4 mL/min/100 g

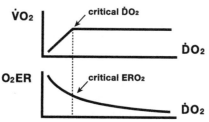

Fig. 4. Relationship between oxygen delivery ($\dot{D}O_2$), tissue oxygen consumption ($\dot{V}O_2$), and oxygen extraction (O_2ER). When $\dot{D}O_2$ decreases, oxygen extraction increases to maintain $\dot{V}O_2$ until a critical point, at which time oxygen consumption falls with further declines in $\dot{D}O_2$. (*Adapted from* Vallet B. Vascular reactivity and tissue oxygenation. Intensive Care Med 1998;24(1):4; with permission; and *Data from* Hungerford JE, Sessa WC, Segal SS. Vasomotor control in arterioles of the mouse cremaster muscle. FASEB J 2000;14(1):197–207.)

body weight. Lieberman and colleagues[41] studied healthy humans, seeking to identify the critical $\dot{D}O_2$ threshold, which they defined as a value below which $\dot{D}O_2$ fails to satisfy metabolic requirements. The investigators concluded that a $\dot{D}O_2$ reduced to 7.3 ± 1.4 mL/kg/min failed to produce evidence of inadequate systemic oxygenation, and thus concluded that the critical $\dot{D}O_2$ threshold must be below this 7.3 mL/kg/min mark.[41] Perhaps more compelling is the findings in a landmark study evaluating septic and nonseptic critically ill patients undergoing withdrawal of life support conducted by Ronco and colleagues.[42] This study reported no difference in critical $\dot{D}O_2$ threshold (3.8 ± 1.5 vs 4.5 ± 1.3 mL/kg/min; $P>.28$) between septic and nonseptic patients, and concluded that the critical $\dot{D}O_2$ value is lower than 4.5 mL/kg/min.

Supply-dependent $\dot{V}O_2$ is closely linked to the concept of redistribution of blood flow. Under normal circumstances blood flow, and thus $\dot{D}O_2$, is organ-matched to metabolic requirements, meaning that each organ receives generally a constant fraction of whole-body $\dot{D}O_2$.[19] When whole-body $\dot{D}O_2$ is compromised, $\dot{D}O_2$ is redistributed to organs unable to increase their O_2ER, such as the brain and heart, which receive proportionately larger amounts of blood flow compared with other organs such as the kidney, gastrointestinal tract, and liver. Redistribution of blood flow tends to enhance the efficiency of oxygen use[43] and maintain homeostasis. Sympathetically mediated vasoconstriction is the mechanism believed to redirect blood flow to metabolically active tissues, preventing the vascular steal phenomenon whereby limited oxygen supply is consumed by tissues with low metabolic demands.[44,45]

MACROCIRCULATION VERSUS MICROCIRCULATION

Ensuring adequate tissue $\dot{D}O_2$ to meet metabolic demands has become a cornerstone of treating critically ill patients. However, current monitoring technology has limited clinical capabilities to global or macro approaches rather than micro approaches, and in many ways has restricted conceptual evolution. At present, the authors are finding the outcomes of critically ill patients to be increasingly tied to function of the microcirculation. Despite monitoring and correction of global hemodynamic variables (ie, macrocirculation), patients develop multiple organ failure and die. Mounting evidence suggests that microcirculatory dysfunction is responsible for poor outcomes attributable to microvascular injury, impaired microvascular control, maldistribution of blood flow leading to tissue oxygen debt, inefficient matching of microvascular oxygen supply to oxygen demand, and impaired oxygen extraction.[3]

Although such global indicators of oxygen balance as CO, mean arterial pressure, SVR, blood gases, $\dot{D}O_2$, and $\dot{V}O_2$ provide useful information on the whole-body state of the cardiovascular system, these parameters fail to provide insight into the state of the microcirculation. Hence, given the current dearth of monitoring and treatment capabilities, microcirculatory abnormalities are underappreciated and undertreated. Developing technologies such as orthogonal polarization spectral imaging, sidestream dark-field imaging, and laser Doppler flowmetry do allow bedside evaluation of the microcirculation, but these techniques are not commonly used as monitoring modalities in today's intensive care unit. Likewise, treatments selectively targeted to resuscitate the microcirculation (eg, ultrashort-acting β1 blockade, recombinant activated protein C) are in the infant stages of development and testing.[46] Although dispiriting, experts advise: "...treat the macrohemodynamic as soon as possible, but if the patient does not get better, look at the microcirculation and try to resuscitate it!"[46(p6)]

SUMMARY

The microcirculation plays a key role in the balance of oxygen delivery ($\dot{D}o_2$) and consumption ($\dot{V}o_2$). Aerobic metabolism and maintenance of organ homeostasis depend on the body's ability to adequately and efficiently deliver oxygen through microcirculatory blood flow and then, via diffusion, on to the mitochondria for utilization. The complex processes of oxygen transport and utilization involve coordination of the lungs, heart, macrovasculature, and microvasculature, all of which are regulated by central nervous system and regional controls. If treatment directed at global hemodynamic and oxygenation abnormalities does not yield improvement of the patient's condition, clinicians are urged to consider the likely possibility of microcirculatory dysfunction. After years of relying on global measures of hemodynamics and oxygenation to treat critically ill patients, a growing body of evidence suggests expectation of a new arsenal of technologies and treatments oriented toward the microcirculation.

REFERENCES

1. Mohrman DE, Heller JJ. Overview of the cardiovascular system. Cardiovascular physiology. 5th edition. New York: Lange Medical Books/McGraw-Hill; 2003. p. 1–18.
2. Hameed SM, Aird WC, Cohn SM. Oxygen delivery. Crit Care Med 2003;31(Suppl 12): S658–67.
3. Bateman RM, Sharpe MD, Ellis CG. Bench-to-bedside review: microvascular dysfunction in sepsis-hemodynamics, oxygen transport, and nitric oxide. Crit Care 2003;7(5):359–73.
4. De Backer D, Donadello K, Taccone FS, et al. Microcirculatory alterations: potential mechanisms and implications for therapy. Ann Intensive Care 2011;1(1):27.
5. Berne RM, Levy MN. The peripheral circulation and its control. Cardiovascular physiology. 8th edition. St Louis (MO): Mosby; 2001. p. 175–97.
6. Opie LH. Introductory cardiovascular concepts. The heart physiology, from cell to circulation. 3rd edition. Philadelphia: Lippincott-Raven; 1998. p. 3–15.
7. Berne RM, Levy MN. The microcirculation and lymphatics. Cardiovascular physiology. 8th edition. St Louis (MO): Mosby; 2001. p. 155–74.
8. Wagner PD. Determinants of maximal oxygen transport and utilization. Annu Rev Physiol 1996;58:21–50.
9. Mohrman DE, Heller LJ. Cardiovascular physiology. 7th edition. New York: McGraw-Hill Medical; 2010.
10. Groom AC, Ellis CG, Wrigley SJ, et al. Capillary network morphology and capillary flow. Int J Microcirc Clin Exp 1995;15:223–30.

11. Lindbom L, Arfors KE. Mechanisms and site of control for variation in the number of perfused capillaries in skeletal muscle. Int J Microcirc Clin Exp 1985;4(1):19–30.

12. Saldivar E, Cabrales P, Tsai AG, et al. Microcirculatory changes during chronic adaptation to hypoxia. Am J Physiol Heart Circ Physiol 2003;285(5):H2064–71.

13. Hepple RT, Mackinnon SL, Goodman JM, et al. Resistance and aerobic training in older men: effects on VO_2 peak and the capillary supply to skeletal muscle. J Appl Physiol (1985) 1997;82(4):1305–10.

14. Farquhar I, Martin CM, Lam C, et al. Decreased capillary density in vivo in bowel mucosa of rats with normotensive sepsis. J Surg Res 1996;61(1):190–6.

15. Ellis CG, Jagger J, Sharpe M. The microcirculation as a functional system. Crit Care 2005;9(Suppl 4):S3–8.

16. Hungerford JE, Sessa WC, Segal SS. Vasomotor control in arterioles of the mouse cremaster muscle. FASEB J 2000;14(1):197–207.

17. Dietrich HH, Ellsworth ML, Sprague RS, et al. Red blood cell regulation of microvascular tone through adenosine triphosphate. Am J Physiol Heart Circ Physiol 2000;278(4):H1294–8.

18. Ellsworth ML. The red blood cell as an oxygen sensor: what is the evidence? Acta Physiol Scand 2000;168(4):551–9.

19. Vallet B. Vascular reactivity and tissue oxygenation. Intensive Care Med 1998; 24(1):3–11.

20. Sielenkamper AW, Kvietys P, Sibbald W. Microvascular alterations in sepsis. In: Vincent JL, Carlet J, Opal S, editors. The sepsis text. Boston: Kluwer Academic Publishers; 2002. p. 247–70.

21. Darovic GO. Cardiovascular anatomy and physiology. In: Darovic GO, editor. Hemodynamic monitoring invasive and noninvasive clinical application. 3rd edition. Philadelphia: W. B. Saunders; 2002. p. 57–90.

22. Ten VS, Pinsky DJ. Endothelial response to hypoxia: physiologic adaptation and pathologic dysfunction. Curr Opin Crit Care 2002;8(3):242–50.

23. Vallet B. Endothelial cell dysfunction and abnormal tissue perfusion. Crit Care Med 2002;30(Suppl 5):S229–34.

24. Muller MM, Griesmacher A. Markers of endothelial dysfunction. Clin Chem Lab Med 2000;38(2):77–85.

25. Segal SS. Regulation of blood flow in the microcirculation. Microcirculation 2005; 12(1):33–45.

26. Bergfeld GR, Forrester T. Release of ATP from human erythrocytes in response to a brief period of hypoxia and hypercapnia. Cardiovasc Res 1992;26(1):40–7.

27. Ellsworth ML, Forrester T, Ellis CG, et al. The erythrocyte as a regulator of vascular tone. Am J Phys 1995;269(6 Pt 2):H2155–61.

28. Collins DM, McCullough WT, Ellsworth ML. Conducted vascular responses: communication across the capillary bed. Microvasc Res 1998;56(1):43–53.

29. Lipowsky HH. Microvascular rheology and hemodynamics. Microcirculation 2005;12(1):5–15.

30. Baskurt OK, Meiselman HJ. Blood rheology and hemodynamics. Semin Thromb Hemost 2003;29(5):435–50.

31. Barvitenko NN, Aslam M, Filosa J, et al. Tissue oxygen demand in regulation of the behavior of the cells in the vasculature. Microcirculation 2013;20(6):484–501.

32. Baskurt OK, Temiz A, Meiselman HJ. Red blood cell aggregation in experimental sepsis. J Lab Clin Med 1997;130(2):183–90.

33. Darovic GO. Monitoring oxygenation. In: Darovic GO, editor. Hemodynamic monitoring invasive and noninvasive clinical application. 3rd edition. Philadelphia: W. B. Saunders; 2002. p. 263–81.

34. Honig CR, Connett RJ, Gayeski TE. O_2 transport and its interaction with metabolism; a systems view of aerobic capacity. Med Sci Sports Exerc 1992;24(1): 47–53.
35. Mik EG. Special article: measuring mitochondrial oxygen tension: from basic principles to application in humans. Anesth Analg 2013;117(4):834–46.
36. Darovic GO, Zbilut JP. Pulmonary anatomy and physiology. In: Darovic GO, editor. Hemodynamic monitoring: invasive and noninvasive clinical application. 3rd edition. Philadelphia: W.B. Saunders Company; 2002. p. 9–42.
37. Shoemaker WC. Relation of oxygen transport patterns to the pathophysiology and therapy of shock states. Intensive Care Med 1987;13(4):230–43.
38. Schlichtig R, Klions HA, Kramer DJ, et al. Hepatic dysoxia commences during O_2 supply dependence. J Appl Physiol (1985) 1992;72(4):1499–505.
39. Brealey D, Singer M. Tissue oxygenation in sepsis. Sepsis 1998;2:291–302.
40. Maruyama R, Fukuda Y. Regulation of oxygen delivery and consumption in anesthetized rats during acute hypoxia. JPN J Physiol 1994;44(5):489–500.
41. Lieberman JA, Weiskopf RB, Kelley SD, et al. Critical oxygen delivery in conscious humans is less than 7.3 ml O_2 x kg(-1) x min(-1). Anesthesiology 2000;92(2):407–13.
42. Ronco JJ, Fenwick JC, Tweeddale MG, et al. Identification of the critical oxygen delivery for anaerobic metabolism in critically ill septic and nonseptic humans. JAMA 1993;270(14):1724–30.
43. Romand JA, Attewell JV, Pinsky MR. Increases in peripheral oxygen demand affect blood flow distribution in hemorrhaged dogs. Am J Respir Crit Care Med 1996;153(1):203–10.
44. Samsel RW, Schumacker PT. Systemic hemorrhage augments local O_2 extraction in canine intestine. J Appl Physiol (1985) 1994;77(5):2291–8.
45. Pinsky MR, Schlichtig R. Regional oxygen delivery in oxygen supply-dependent states. Intensive Care Med 1990;16(Suppl 2):S169–71.
46. Donati A, Domizi R, Damiani E, et al. From macrohemodynamic to the microcirculation. Crit Care Res Pract 2013;2013:892710.

The Physiologic Role of Erythrocytes in Oxygen Delivery and Implications for Blood Storage

Penelope S. Benedik, PhD, RN, CRNA, RRT[a],*,
Shannan K. Hamlin, PhD, RN, ACNP-BC, AGACNP-BC, CCRN[b]

KEYWORDS

- Red blood cell • Nitric oxide • Oxygen transport • Hemoglobin • Storage lesion

KEY POINTS

- Erythrocytes are complex, metabolically active cells that exert a powerful influence on the microvascular circulation.
- Along with transporting oxygen bound to hemoglobin molecules, red blood cells act as local oxygen sensors, triggering the release of vasodilatory mediators so that vessels dilate when oxygen levels are low.
- There is some evidence that an erythrocyte storage lesion uncouples deoxygenated hemoglobin from vasodilator release, and that this phenomenon negatively impacts outcome in trauma patients.
- Cryopreservation—freezing to temperatures as low as −80° Celsius– appears to preserve the more sensitive physiologic functions of stored erythrocytes.

INTRODUCTION

Erythrocytes containing hemoglobin (Hb) were identified as the primary oxygen transport mechanism in humans more than 100 years ago.[1] In clinical practice, the role of red blood cells (RBC) in oxygen delivery is generally defined by evaluating the mass of Hb present and the relationship between dissolved oxygen and Hb saturation. Emphasis is placed on the interaction between the RBC and oxygen at the level of the lung: ventilatory parameters are adjusted with the purpose of improving the

Funding Sources: Nil.
Conflict of Interest: Nil.
[a] Department of Acute and Continuing Care, School of Nursing, University of Texas Health Science Center at Houston, 6901 Bertner Street, SON 682, Houston, TX 77030, USA; [b] Nursing Research and Evidence-Based Practice, Houston Methodist Hospital, 6565 Fannin, MGJ 11-017, Houston, TX 77030, USA
* Corresponding author.
E-mail address: Penelope.S.Benedik@uth.tmc.edu

Crit Care Nurs Clin N Am 26 (2014) 325–335
http://dx.doi.org/10.1016/j.ccell.2014.04.002
0899-5885/14/$ – see front matter © 2014 Elsevier Inc. All rights reserved.

oxygen content of the blood leaving the pulmonary capillary bed. The attention paid to blood flow is also at the organ level: we monitor the cardiac output to describe regional organ and tissue perfusion.

This concept of oxygen delivery is clearly focused on a whole body or "macro" view. Current critical care interventions are very effective at adjusting the components of oxygen delivery:

Oxygen (O_2) delivery = O_2 Content (mL O_2/dL blood) $\times$ Cardiac Output (L/min)

O_2 Content = O_2 Bound to Hb + Dissolved O_2

Dissolved O_2 (mL O_2/dL blood) = Arterial P_{O_2} (mm Hg) $\times$ 0.003 mL O_2/mm Hg P_{O_2}/dL blood

Bound O_2 = 1.36 mL O_2/g Hb /dL blood $\times$ Grams of Hb $\times$ % Hb saturated with O_2

Oxygen delivery depends on many factors including, but not limited to, the ability of the right ventricle to deliver an adequate blood supply to the pulmonary capillary bed, adequate diffusion of oxygen across the alveolar capillary membrane, the ability of the left ventricle to move oxygenated blood out of the central circulation, and notably a vascular response that permits flow of oxygenated blood to a variety of tissue beds with different metabolic needs.

Oxygen content comprises dissolved oxygen (Pa_{O_2}) and oxygen bound to Hb. Hb-bound oxygen therefore depends on the mass of available Hb, the intrinsic carrying capacity of Hb, and what part of the hemoglobin's binding capacity is being used. The carrying capacity of Hb depends on several factors including the type of Hb present and a variety of environmental factors (pH, P_{CO_2}, temperature, chemical milieu), some of which can be adjusted clinically.

More recently attention has focused on the physical properties and responsiveness of the erythrocyte to its local environment and the dynamics of its movement through the microcirculation.[2] This article reviews the functional anatomy and applied physiology of the erythrocyte and the microcirculation with an emphasis on how erythrocytes modulate microvascular function. Also briefly discussed are the effects of cell storage on the metabolic functions of the erythrocyte.

HB IN AN ERYTHROCYTE ACTIVELY RESPONDS TO ITS LOCAL ENVIRONMENT

RBCs have several features that serve to improve their ability to transport oxygen between the lung and peripheral tissue beds. The biconcave shape maximizes the surface area of the cell and decreases the diffusion distance for oxygen and carbon dioxide. The RBC membrane is deformable, allowing it to squeeze through vessels narrower in diameter than itself, although this flexibility lessens in the presence of hypoxia and during storage.

Erythrocytes are packed with Hb. Each RBC contains between 200 and 300 million Hb molecules and each Hb binds up to four oxygen molecules.[3] Hemoglobin wafts between a relaxed (oxygenated) and tense (deoxygenated) state in response to the current dissolved oxygen tension. Some Hb molecules are actually embedded in the RBC membrane and these Hb molecules have the potential to act as oxygen sensors. Although binding of the first oxygen molecule to Hb is difficult, each successive binding slightly alters the globin chains such that each successive oxygen binding becomes easier. These binding characteristics explain the steep segment of the sigmoid-shaped oxyhemoglobin dissociation curve.

High dissolved oxygen levels, high pH, and low $Paco_2$ favor oxygen uptake by Hb in the pulmonary capillary bed, whereas low Pao_2, low pH, and a high $Paco_2$ favor oxygen release at the tissues. The latter event, in which slight hypercarbia and acidosis favor oxygen unloading at the tissue bed, makes physiologic sense and is known as the Bohr effect. Commonly, clinical focus has been on oxygen movement between Hb saturations of 100% and 70% (the typical arterial to mixed venous gradient). However, oxygen transfer at the tissue bed occurs at much lower partial pressures of oxygen and oxygen saturation, suggesting that low tissue Po_2 influences both Hb and RBC behavior.[4]

Beyond oxygen transport, erythrocytes have significant metabolic functions. The Hb molecule contributes substantively to buffering the hydrogen ions (H^+) formed by the hydration of CO_2 in the cell. Thus, slight acidosis may be noted in patients with severe anemia whose buffering capacity is hampered by low Hb levels. Additionally, both adenosine triphosphate (ATP) and nitric oxide (NO) synthesis occur within the RBC. It has been suggested that the RBC senses tissue hypoxia and responds to it by releasing vasodilators that act on local smooth muscle to increase flow to the "relatively" hypoxic area.[5]

THE MICROCIRCULATION IS DESIGNED TO RESPOND TO LOCAL TISSUE NEEDS

The microcirculation represents blood flow through the smallest blood vessels, typically those vessels that are embedded inside tissue beds. These vessels include the precapillary arterioles, capillaries, and postcapillary venules.[6] Arterioles average 100 μm in diameter and contain smooth muscle, whereas capillary vessels range in diameter from 5 to 10 μm and are formed by only endothelial cells and basement membrane. Autoregulation, and therefore local control of tissue perfusion, occurs at the arteriolar level and smooth muscle here is highly responsive to sympathetic stimulation, NO, endothelin-1, and other chemical mediators.

The capillary bed is a delicate structure comprised of a large number of very small vessels with a high cross-sectional surface area. Diffusion distance is the smallest here because of the thinness of the capillary membrane, although increases in capillary density may contribute to an increased transfer of oxygen in this area. Venules are high-capacity, low-pressure, and thin-walled vessels that exhibit increases in smooth muscle as they become larger. Not all vessels in the microcirculation are always perfused; previously closed vessels may be recruited during periods of increased metabolic demand.

Oxygen diffuses not only out of capillaries but also extensively out of arterioles and to some degree out of venules. These oxygen molecules are destined to supply neighboring cells and/or other vessels in close proximity and seem to be substantively consumed by the metabolically active muscular cells in the arteriolar wall.[4] It is estimated that approximately two-thirds of the oxygen loss from the blood occurs across the arterioles and one-third from the capillaries. Oxygen gradients in the microcirculation are also altered by the tissue metabolic needs: increases in metabolism create large gradients when compared with the resting state.

CAPILLARY ENDOTHELIAL CELLS CREATE A METABOLIC LINK BETWEEN THE TISSUE AND THE BLOOD

The endothelial cells that line the microcirculation are metabolically active and form the link between the blood and the tissue bed. Although functions common to all endothelial cells include modulating coagulation and inflammatory processes, there is significant variability in endothelial cell function across different tissue types. The extent of endothelial participation in the regulation of tissue blood flow has led its role to be characterized as a "distributed signaling network."[7] Capillary endothelial cells respond chemically to mechanical deformation and/or hypoxia by generating NO, endothelin-1, ATP, and other mediators that act to modulate flow locally and at distant vascular walls.

ATP molecules are produced by the erythrocytes primarily when they are exposed to low levels of dissolved oxygen in the vascular lumen (Po_2 approximately 22–24 mm Hg).[8,9] The released ATP elicits a vasodilator response locally and in the surrounding microcirculation that occurs in about 0.5 second.[10] It seems that the low-oxygen induced ATP release is triggered by the desaturation of RBC-membrane bound Hb molecules; that is, structural change in these deoxygenated Hb molecules elicits a structural deformation in the RBC membrane and subsequent ATP release.[11] This type of erythrocyte-derived ATP is thought to be an important regulator of oxygen supply to working skeletal muscle; exercising muscle extracts relatively more oxygen and deoxygenates Hb, which triggers ATP release and vasodilation.[12,13] It has been suggested that impaired release of ATP from erythrocytes may contribute to impaired muscle perfusion.[11]

Once released from the RBC, ATP interacts with purinergic receptors on vascular endothelial cells to release vasodilators, the most important of which is NO. Other vasodilators released after purinergic stimulation include prostaglandin I_2 (prostacyclin) and epoxyeicosatrienoic acid. Released ATP subsequently forms cyclic AMP, which is the "second messenger" that triggers the downstream release of vasodilators. Inhibiting cyclic AMP breakdown would allow the accumulation of cyclic AMP and improved vasodilation. Cyclic AMP is broken down by a specific phosphodiesterase in the subtype 3 family. In fact, phosphodiesterase subtype 3A and 3B have been identified in this process with the localization of these phosphodiesterase subtypes in the vascular smooth muscle of patients with type 2 diabetes.[14]

Vascular endothelial cells contain NO synthase, an enzyme responsible for regulating the production of NO. The classic pathway for NO formation is oxygen dependent. However, an oxygen-independent pathway to NO formation has been suggested that could reduce nitrate → nitrite → NO in either acidic or hypoxic environments, enhancing vasodilation under these conditions.[7] Deoxygenated Hb binds nitrate and reduces it to NO, a useful effect in situations of compromised tissue blood flow or oxygenation (**Fig. 1**).

These mechanisms form the basis for impaired vasodilation in patients with type 2 diabetes mellitus. In this disease, erythrocyte defects have been linked to decreased ATP release and lack of vasodilation when exposed to low oxygen levels.[11] Additionally, chronic exposure to increased insulin levels that precede clinically demonstrable hyperglycemia seem to elicit a similar dysfunction of the ATP-vasodilator signaling pathway. These effects are thought to contribute to the adverse effects of diabetes and prediabetes on the microvasculature. Defects in erythrocyte ATP release have also been found in cystic fibrosis and idiopathic pulmonary hypertension.

HB IS A HETEROGENEOUS AND SENSITIVE MOLECULE

The type of Hb present affects the kinetics of oxygen binding and oxygen release at the tissue beds. In adults, approximately 95% of Hb is HbA, which has the binding characteristics previously described. A newborn has 50% to 95% HbF, which has a very high affinity for oxygen and decreases oxygen release at the tissue; adults

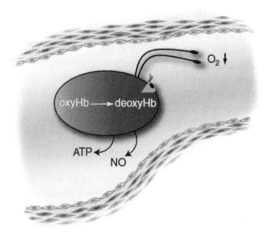

Fig. 1. This graphic illustrates that red blood cells sense local hypoxia via cellular membrane-embeded hemoglobin. Deoxyhemoglobin seems to trigger the release of ATP and NO, which increase vessel diameter, improving local blood flow to match oxygen demand to oxygen delivery. (*From* Jensen FB. The dual roles of red blood cells in tissue oxygen delivery: oxygen carriers and regulators of local blood flow. J Exp Biol 2009;212(Pt 21):3389; with permission.)

generally exhibit less than 1% HbF. Up to 3.5% of adult Hb may be HbA_2, which has a poor affinity for carrying oxygen.[3] Patients with β-thalassemia produce both HbA_2 and HbF, whereas homozygotes for sickle cell disease have an increased Hb affinity for oxygen. Glycated Hb (HbA_{1c}) is a form of Hb known to be associated with long-term high glucose levels. Increased HbA_{1c} (>7%) shifts the oxyhemoglobin dissociation curve to the left, reducing hemoglobin's ability to release oxygen at the tissue beds.[15]

Methemoglobin is formed when the ferrous iron (Fe^{++}) in Hb is oxidized to ferric iron (Fe^{+++}). Methemoglobin cannot bind oxygen and shifts the oxyhemoglobin curve to the left while reducing the oxygen carrying capacity of the molecule. Methemoglobin may be induced by drugs, such as prilocaine (including the use of EMLA, a lidocaine-prilocaine topical), benzocaine, nitrates (inhaled amyl or butyl nitrate, nitroglycerin, nitroprusside), dapsone, and others.[16,17]

Both carbon monoxide and NO can combine with Hb. Unfortunately, the affinity of Hb for carbon monoxide is more than 200 times greater than the Hb affinity for oxygen. In the presence of carbon monoxide, oxygen loses the competition for binding sites on Hb and carboxyhemoglobin forms. Depending on the degree of carbon monoxide exposure, the oxygen-carrying capacity of Hb may be substantially reduced while the dissolved oxygen levels are normal. In the presence of carboxyhemoglobin, the Po_2 must decrease to a much lower level for the release of oxygen, making tissue hypoxia more likely.[18]

Other local environmental influences on hemoglobin's affinity for oxygen deserve some remarks. Increases in the hydrogen ion concentration, partial pressure of carbon dioxide, temperature, and concentration of 2,3-diphosphoglycerate (2,3-DPG) decrease hemoglobin's affinity for oxygen, whereas decreasing the same factors has the opposite effect. The substrate 2,3-DPG is produced in large quantities in the RBC and is increased in anemia and at altitude, conditions in which tissue oxygenation may be compromised. Increases in tissue metabolism that lead to hypercarbia or acidosis also serve to improve oxygen release at the tissue and are associated with a right shift in the oxyhemoglobin dissociation curve.

HB CARRIES AND RELEASES THE POTENT VASODILATOR NO

NO interacts with Hb in two ways: NO may bind to the heme group on Hb (NO-Hb) or NO may react with the amino acid cysteine found in the globin chains to form a nitrosothiol (SNO-Hb). Nitrosohemoglobin more commonly occurs in arterial blood, whereas in venous blood NO is bound to heme. The transition to deoxyhemoglobin during RBC passage through a tissue bed releases the cysteinyl-bound NO, allowing it to diffuse from the RBC as a local vasodilator (**Fig. 2**).[3] This suggests that Hb desaturation, not low dissolved oxygen (Po_2), is coupled to the NO component of the vasodilator response.

STORING ERYTHROCYTES ALTERS THEIR OPTIMAL FUNCTION

Erythrocytes are delicate and metabolically active cells with a life span of approximately 120 days. This reminds us that even when the freshest possible blood is delivered to the patient, the delivered cells are in various stages of maturity. Erythrocytes are subjected to storage in an artificial milieu after donation; it is well known that storage attenuates the cells' ability to function normally after transfusion. The changes that occur in stored blood are characterized as a RBC "storage lesion." The lesion begins

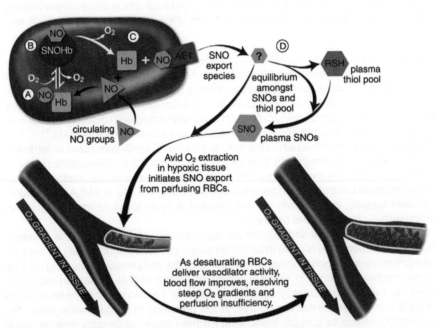

Fig. 2. Metabolic responses of the erythrocyte to local oxygen levels are translated into vascular responses by the activity of NO. RBC-bound hemoglobin wafts between its oxygenated state (*B*) in which NO is carried or stored as nitrosothiols and its deoxygenated state (*A*) in which NO is easily released. When the blood-to-tissue oxygen diffusion gradient favors oxygen release, released NO acts locally to vasodilate the immediate area. NO groups are also carried in the plasma. (*C*) Nitric oxide processing couples vessel tone to tissue Po_2, creating a hypoxic vasodilation in order to match blood flow to regional needs. (*D*) and as parts of other cellular elements. AE1, a membrane protein that transfers NO released from hemoglobin to outside the cell; RSH, a thiol-(sulfur)-containing protein or peptide; SNO, S-nitrosothiols. (*From* Doctor A, Spinella P. Effect of processing and storage on red blood cell function in vivo. Semin Perinatol 2012;36:251; with permission.)

to appear after about 7 days of storage and continues to increase thereafter.[19] These structural and physiologic changes are summarized in **Table 1** and **Fig. 3**.

DOES RBC STORAGE TIME MATTER?

Erythrocyte storage lesions may be time-dependent: in some studies, fresh RBCs (from 0 to 4 days of storage) are associated with fewer adverse effects than older RBCs (21–42 days).[20,21] In one study, muscle tissue oxygenation and perfused capillary density were negatively associated with increased RBC storage age, suggesting that fresh blood has immediate benefits.[21] However, several studies have reported no differences in outcomes between patients transfused with fresh versus old blood.[22,23] In a randomized controlled trial in very low birth weight premature infants by Fergusson and colleagues,[23] fresh blood had a mean age of 5.1 days, whereas the control group received blood with a mean age of 14.6 days, blood that would not be considered "old" by some authors. In a retrospective cohort study in cardiac surgery

---

Table 1
Physiologic effects of processing and storing erythrocytes

Storage Effect	Potential Outcome
Increased potassium	Risk of hyperkalemia
Increased lactate	Initial acidosis
Citrate toxicity	Hypocalcemia, hypomagnesemia
RBC lysis and cell death	Increased free hemoglobin
Hemolysis increases significantly by storage day 10–12	Increased unbound iron → increases infection risk
	Decreased oxygen delivery
Decreased 2,3-DPG	Left shift the oxyhemoglobin dissociation curve with limited oxygen unloading
Decreased ATP and NO	Limits passage through microcirculation
Loss of cell deformability with formation of abnormal cell shape	Increases cell aggregation and adhesion to endothelium
Release of soluble lipids	Facilitates thrombin formation
Accumulation of	Febrile transfusion reactions
Interleukin-6	Downregulation of recipient immune function
Interleukin-8	
Phospholipase A_2	Increased cancer recurrence
Superoxide anions	Increased postoperative infection rates
Decreased tumor necrosis factor-α	Transfusion-related immune modulation
	Transfusion-related acute lung injury

Data from Refs.[20,24–26]

---

patients by Voorhuis and colleagues,[22] the median storage age was 13 ± 2 days for "young" blood and 21 ± 5 days for "older" blood. Patients who were transfused with more than 7 units were excluded from analysis. In a blinded, randomized controlled trial of medical and surgical intensive care patients, Kor and colleagues[27] reported that transfusion of just 1 unit of fresh blood (median storage, 4 days) versus 1 unit of standard blood (median storage, 26.5 days) resulted in no differences in pulmonary, immunologic, or coagulation outcomes. In a 2013 retrospective analysis, Middelburg and colleagues[28] provide a thoughtful analysis that demonstrated how the design and statistical choices made by researchers can significantly alter reported results.

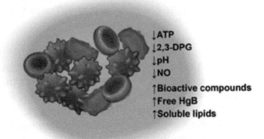

↓ATP
↓2,3-DPG
↓pH
↓NO
↑Bioactive compounds
↑Free HgB
↑Soluble lipids

Fig. 3. The effects of storage on erythrocytes include detrimental decreases in ATP, 2,3-DPG, pH, and NO and increases in bioactive compounds, Hb, and soluble lipids. See text for details. (*From* Koch CG, Figueroa PI, Li L, et al. Red blood cell storage: how long is too long? Ann Thorac Surg 2013;96:1896; with permission.)

HOW DOES STORAGE AFFECT THE ERYTHROCYTE?

When trauma patients are transfused with 3 or more units of blood older than 14 days versus fresh blood, even when controlling for the degree of trauma and demographics, the odds of mortality, acute kidney injury, pneumonia, and respiratory distress syndrome increase.[29] It has been suggested that storage uncouples the intimate relationship between deoxygenated Hb and both ATP and NO release so that old blood is less able to regulate flow in the microcirculation.[19,21] This metabolic function of the erythrocyte may play a more important role in an acute trauma victim than in other medical conditions.

Blood transfusion can be thought of as a "liquid organ" transplant. This creates an immunologic event that includes the release of cytokines and complement. Leukocytes produce proinflammatory cytokines that contribute to systemic inflammation and a higher risk of bacterial infection. Complement activation occurs even in leukocyte-reduced transfusion products because of the presence of complement in plasma and by activating complement in the nondepleted leukocytes. Transfusing erythrocytes can elicit the formation of complement-activating antigen-antibody complexes. Both antigen-antibody complexes and C-reactive protein are formed during erythrocyte storage. Thus, it has been hypothesized that older blood is more inflammatory than fresh blood. This is one mechanism hypothesized to explain transfusion-related acute lung injury.[19,24]

Although blood storage up to 42 days is medically acceptable, transfusion (especially massive transfusion) of blood products older than 14, 19, 21, 28, or 30 days generally increases morbidity and mortality (see Koch and colleagues[20]). Some authors recommend limiting RBC storage to 14 days, whereas others believe that adverse effects of transfusion are more influenced by the total amount of RBCs delivered rather than the storage duration.[22] Research in this area is equivocal and ongoing, including efforts to improve the current management of the blood supply.

BIOPRESERVATION OF ERYTHROCYTES

Blood preservation depends on maintaining the functional efficacy of the RBC: the integrity of the RBC membrane, the Hb molecules, and cellular energetics must all be preserved.[30] Defects in any of these areas result in hemolysis and a less than normal RBC functional lifespan. Hypothermia (temperatures in the 1°C–6°C range) reduces cellular reaction rates but incompletely. Therefore, continuing cellular metabolism depletes ATP and 2,3-DPG and lowers pH because of the accumulation of lactic acid. These biochemical changes decrease RBC deformability and adhesiveness while increasing internal cell viscosity and hemolysis. To help overcome these effects, additive solutions contain adenine and glucose along with the cell membrane stabilizers, mannitol and citrate. Leukocyte reduction removes highly metabolic cells and minimizes glucose consumption. However, despite these efforts, by the end of the 42-day shelf-life, only 75% of the RBCs are viable, and this minimum accepted viability does not reflect the cells' in vivo performance.[31]

Recent studies have demonstrated that cryopreservation of erythrocytes may be effective in preserving the more sensitive physiologic functions of stored RBCs.[32] Cryopreservation entails freezing and storing blood products at temperatures low enough to suppress molecular motion and completely halt metabolic reactions (from −80°C to −150°C).[30] Erythrocyte membranes, Hb structure, and cellular metabolism seem to be unaffected by extended storage in this state. Strict attention must be paid to achieve optimal cooling and thawing rates and to the solutions used during cryopreservation (see Scott and coworkers[30]).

Hampton and Schreiber,[32] in a review of near infrared spectroscopy, provided some compelling graphical data that a significant improvement in tissue oxygenation occurred after administration of cryopreserved versus standard blood in a trauma population. Cryopreserved blood products are used extensively in military operations and may become a significant resource for the long-term storage of rare blood type components.[33]

SUMMARY

Erythrocytes are complex, metabolically active cells that exert a powerful influence on the microvascular circulation. Along with transporting oxygen bound to Hb molecules, RBCs act as local oxygen sensors, triggering the release of vasodilatory mediators so that vessels dilate when oxygen levels are low. The sensitivity of this system seems to be harmed by lengthy blood storage, making older RBCs less effective at improving tissue oxygenation. Cryopreservation, an alternative to standard hypothermic blood banking storage techniques, may become a useful adjunct to more physiologically effective hemotherapy in practice.

REFERENCES

1. Weber RE, Campbell KL. Temperature dependence of haemoglobin-oxygen affinity in heterothermic vertebrates: mechanisms and biological significance. Acta Physiol (Oxf) 2011;202(3):549–62.
2. Baskurt OK, Meiselman HJ. Blood rheology and hemodynamics. Semin Thromb Hemost 2003;29(5):435–50.
3. Thomas C, Lumb A. Physiology of haemoglobin. Cont Educ Anaesth Crit Care Pain 2013;12(5):251–6.
4. Pittman RN. Oxygen gradients in the microcirculation. Acta Physiol (Oxf) 2011; 202(3):311–22.
5. Jensen FB. The dual roles of red blood cells in tissue oxygen delivery: oxygen carriers and regulators of local blood flow. J Exp Biol 2009;212(Pt 21):3387–93.
6. Ekbal NJ, Dyson A, Black C, et al. Monitoring tissue perfusion, oxygenation, and metabolism in critically ill patients. Chest 2013;143(6):1799–808.

7. Somani A, Steiner ME, Hebbel RP. The dynamic regulation of microcirculatory conduit function: features relevant to transfusion medicine. Transfus Apher Sci 2010;43(1):61–8.

8. Sprague RS, Ellsworth ML. Erythrocyte-derived ATP and perfusion distribution: role of intracellular and intercellular communication. Microcirculation 2012; 19(5):430–9.

9. Sridharan M, Sprague RS, Adderley SP, et al. Diamide decreases deformability of rabbit erythrocytes and attenuates low oxygen tension-induced ATP release. Exp Biol Med (Maywood) 2010;235(9):1142–8.

10. Dietrich HH, Ellsworth ML, Sprague RS, et al. Red blood cell regulation of microvascular tone through adenosine triphosphate. Am J Physiol Heart Circ Physiol 2000;278(4):H1294–8.

11. Sprague RS, Bowles EA, Achilleus D, et al. Erythrocytes as controllers of perfusion distribution in the microvasculature of skeletal muscle. Acta Physiol (Oxf) 2011;202(3):285–92.

12. Gonzalez-Alonso J, Mortensen SP, Dawson EA, et al. Erythrocytes and the regulation of human skeletal muscle blood flow and oxygen delivery: role of erythrocyte count and oxygenation state of haemoglobin. J Physiol 2006;572(Pt 1): 295–305.

13. Richardson RS. Oxygen transport and utilization: an integration of the muscle systems. Adv Physiol Educ 2003;27(1–4):183–91.

14. Sprague RS, Bowles EA, Achilleus D, et al. A selective phosphodiesterase 3 inhibitor rescues low PO2-induced ATP release from erythrocytes of humans with type 2 diabetes: implication for vascular control. Am J Physiol Heart Circ Physiol 2011;301(6):H2466–72.

15. Pu LJ, Shen Y, Lu L, et al. Increased blood glycohemoglobin A1c levels lead to overestimation of arterial oxygen saturation by pulse oximetry in patients with type 2 diabetes. Cardiovasc Diabetol 2012;11:110.

16. Hunter L, Gordge L, Dargan PI, et al. Methaemoglobinaemia associated with the use of cocaine and volatile nitrites as recreational drugs: a review. Br J Clin Pharmacol 2011;72(1):18–26.

17. do Nascimento TS, Pereira RO, de Mello HL, et al. Methemoglobinemia: from diagnosis to treatment. Rev Bras Anestesiol 2008;58(6):651–64.

18. Toffaletti J, Zijlstra WG. Misconceptions in reporting oxygen saturation. Anesth Analg 2007;105(Suppl 6):S5–9.

19. Weinberg JA, Barnum SR, Patel RP. Red blood cell age and potentiation of transfusion-related pathology in trauma patients. Transfusion 2011;51(4): 867–73.

20. Koch CG, Figueroa PI, Li L, et al. Red blood cell storage: how long is too long? Ann Thorac Surg 2013;96(5):1894–9.

21. Weinberg JA, MacLennan PA, Vandromme-Cusick MJ, et al. The deleterious effect of red blood cell storage on microvascular response to transfusion. J Trauma Acute Care Surg 2013;75(5):807–12.

22. Voorhuis FT, Dieleman JM, de Vooght KM, et al. Storage time of red blood cell concentrates and adverse outcomes after cardiac surgery: a cohort study. Ann Hematol 2013;92(12):1701–6.

23. Fergusson DA, Hebert P, Hogan DL, et al. Effect of fresh red blood cell transfusions on clinical outcomes in premature, very low-birth-weight infants: the ARIPI randomized trial. JAMA 2012;308(14):1443–51.

24. Doctor A, Spinella P. Effect of processing and storage on red blood cell function in vivo. Semin Perinatol 2012;36(4):248–59.

25. Isbister JP. Hemorheological considerations in stored blood transfusion. In: Baskurt OK, Hardeman MR, Rampling MW, et al, editors. Handbook of hemorheology and hemodynamics. Amsterdam: IOS Press; 2007. p. 228–41.

26. Rajashekharaiah V, Koshy AA, Koushik AK, et al. The efficacy of erythrocytes isolated from blood stored under blood bank conditions. Transfus Apher Sci 2012; 47(3):359–64.

27. Kor DJ, Kashyap R, Weiskopf RB, et al. Fresh red blood cell transfusion and short-term pulmonary, immunologic, and coagulation status: a randomized clinical trial. Am J Respir Crit Care Med 2012;185(8):842–50.

28. Middelburg RA, van de Watering LM, Briet E, et al. Storage time of red blood cells and mortality of transfusion recipients. Transfus Med Rev 2013;27(1):36–43.

29. Weinberg JA, McGwin G Jr, Marques MB, et al. Transfusions in the less severely injured: does age of transfused blood affect outcomes? J Trauma 2008;65(4): 794–8.

30. Scott KL, Lecak J, Acker JP. Biopreservation of red blood cells: past, present, and future. Transfus Med Rev 2005;19(2):127–42.

31. Hogman CF, Meryman HT. Storage parameters affecting red blood cell survival and function after transfusion. Transfus Med Rev 1999;13(4):275–96.

32. Hampton DA, Schreiber MA. Near infrared spectroscopy: clinical and research uses. Transfusion 2013;53(Suppl 1):52S–8S.

33. Holovati JL, Hannon JL, Gyongyossy-Issa MI, et al. Blood preservation workshop: new and emerging trends in research and clinical practice. Transfus Med Rev 2009;23(1):25–41.

Basic Concepts of Hemorheology in Microvascular Hemodynamics

 CrossMark

Shannan K. Hamlin, PhD, RN, ACNP-BC, AGACNP-BC, CCRN[a],*,
Penelope S. Benedik, PhD, RN, CRNA, RRT[b]

KEYWORDS

- Hemorheology • Microvascular • Hemodynamics • Viscosity
- Erythrocyte deformability • Erythrocyte aggregation • Blood flow • Tissue perfusion

KEY POINTS

- Blood rheology, or hemorheology, involves the science of flow and deformation behavior of blood and its formed elements (ie, erythrocytes, leukocytes, platelets).
- It is well known that the adequacy of blood flow to meet metabolic demands through large circulatory vessels depends highly on vascular control mechanisms.
- The extent to which rheologic properties of blood contribute to vascular flow resistance, particularly in the microcirculation, is becoming more appreciated.
- Current evidence suggests that microvascular blood flow is determined by local vessel resistance and hemorheologic factors such as blood viscosity, erythrocyte deformability, and erythrocyte aggregation. Such knowledge of the behavior of microvascular blood flow promises to be a significant benefit for clinicians who care for patients with hemodynamic alterations.

INTRODUCTION

The function of blood is to deliver oxygen and nutrients to every cell in the body and to remove waste products. To accomplish this, blood must transverse a complicated vascular network comprising vessel diameters ranging from 3 cm to 5 μm at a circulating flow rate sufficient to meet the metabolic demands of organs and tissue beds. The flow behavior of blood is a major determinant in oxygen delivery and tissue perfusion, and depends on the driving pressure generated by the heart, vascular hindrance (ie, diameter and length), and the rheologic properties of the blood. For centuries,

Funding Sources: Nil.
Conflict of Interest: Nil.
[a] Nursing Research and Evidence-Based Practice, Houston Methodist Hospital, 6565 Fannin, MGJ 11-017, Houston, TX 77030, USA; [b] UT Health School of Nursing, University of Texas Health Science Center at Houston, 6901 Bertner Street, Room 682, Houston, TX 77030, USA
* Corresponding author.
E-mail address: SHamlin@HoustonMethodist.org

scientists have investigated the vascular control mechanisms responsible for delivering oxygenated blood to tissues and organs. However, within the past 3 decades scientists have taken a strong interest in improving our understanding of blood rheology and tissue perfusion under dynamic conditions in the macrocirculation and microcirculation. Although global oxygen transport parameters such as cardiac output, oxygen delivery, and oxygen consumption are useful in determining the status of the cardiovascular system (macrocirculation), these parameters fail to provide insight into the state of the microcirculation, which is vital to tissue and organ function. In fact, hemorheologic disorders are among the most significant microcirculatory disturbances in the pathogenesis of hemorrhagic and septic shock. As such, it is important for clinical care staff to have an understanding of blood rheology, or hemorheology. This article discusses the basic concepts involved in hemorheology as it relates to blood-flow resistance in the microcirculation.

COMPOSITION OF BLOOD

Blood is a 2-phase fluid comprising various cells (ie, erythrocytes, leukocytes, platelets) and a liquid phase (ie, plasma) in which the cellular components of blood are suspended. The plasma is a complex solution of various materials (ie, proteins, lipoproteins, and metabolites) that make up approximately 9% of plasma by weight, the rest being water.[1] Under normal conditions plasma viscosity is generally thought to play a minimal role in flow resistance at the macrovascular or microvascular level. However, under pathologic conditions such as acute-phase reactions (ie, infection, postsurgical trauma), the increase in plasma proteins, especially fibrinogen, will contribute significantly to the nonspecific increase of plasma viscosity, with deleterious effects on blood flow in all circulatory vessels but especially those of the microcirculation.[1,2]

In relation to flow behavior, the red blood cells (erythrocytes) are the most prominent and influential component of blood at all levels of the circulatory system, either under bulk flow conditions in large blood vessels or in the microcirculation.[1,3] Their primary role is to facilitate the transport of oxygen and carbon dioxide to and from tissues and organs of the body. Erythrocytes are a single type consisting of a membranous sack containing a concentrated hemoglobin solution. For erythrocytes to survive in the harsh environment of the circulation, they must be able to rapidly undergo deformability and have extreme membrane stability when exposed to hemodynamic shear.[4] An erythrocyte will transverse the circulation more than 1000 times each day during its average 120-day life-span.[4]

Involved in defense against infection, white blood cells (leukocytes), on the other hand, are made up of several distinct varieties (ie, monocytes, granulocytes, and lymphocytes), all containing complicated interiors of organelles and a nucleus suspended in a viscous cytoplasm. Leukocytes play a small role in determining the viscosity of whole blood (ie, macrocirculation) because their number and volume concentration are much smaller than those of erythrocytes.[1] However, leukocytes play a major role in determining flow through the microcirculation for 2 reasons: (1) their internal content has greater viscosity and elasticity than that of the erythrocyte, and (2) all varieties of leukocytes are larger and stiffer, with slower deformability than the erythrocyte.[1] Leukocytes are slow and move erratically, which can delay and modify the capillary transit of the erythrocyte and influence microvascular resistance and tissue perfusion.[5]

Finally, platelets are all essentially similar in their composition; they are anucleated and have relatively complex contents of vacuoles and fibers suspended in a viscous cytoplasm. Their role is in hemostasis. Although platelets have a complex internal content with considerable viscosity, they influence neither whole-blood viscosity nor microvascular resistance because of their much smaller size (diameter 2–3 µm) in comparison with erythrocytes or leukocytes. Moreover, their overall volume is even less than that of leukocytes.[1]

PRINCIPLES OF RHEOLOGY

Rheology is the flow and deformation behavior of solids and fluids. Deformation, a critical concept in the understanding of fluid dynamics, is the relative displacement of material (eg, erythrocytes) by the use of force (eg, vessel diameter) such that the deformation is proportional to the applied force; shape recovery occurs when the force is removed with a time constraint of 0.1 second.[2,3] The force or stress applied per unit area is considered when discussing the degree of deformation, and involves (1) shear stress when the force is acting parallel to the surface and (2) normal stress when the force is acting perpendicular to the surface, also known as the pressure in a fluid.[2] Shear rate is the degree of deformation.

Early flow-mechanics experiments conducted in the nineteenth century by the French physiologist Poiseuille showed that resistance to fluid flow in a pipe depended on flow conditions when the pipe was a constant diameter and length. In slow-flow states the pressure drop, which is a reflection of the resistance to flow, is proportional to the speed of flow.[6] The liquid particles move smoothly and orderly in adjacent planes parallel to the tube wall (laminar flow), which signifies the absence of variations. As the flow rate increases, the flow becomes irregular and chaotic (turbulent flow) with the degree of turbulence proportional to the increase in flow rate. Under turbulent flow conditions, the pressure drop is proportional to the square of the flow rate; therefore, resistance to flow is greater than occurs in laminar flow states.[2]

The fluid of laminar flow states are homogeneous (Newtonian fluid), such as water, in which the shear rate is proportional to the shear stress as opposed to a suspension such as blood (non-Newtonian fluid) wherein the shear rate and stress are not proportional.[6] Fluid flow varies in accordance with the nature of the fluid, known as viscosity or the inherent resistance to flow. Flow rate varies inversely with viscosity.

HEMORHEOLOGY

Blood rheology, or hemorheology, involves the flow and deformation behavior of blood and its formed elements (ie, erythrocytes, leukocytes, platelets).[7] As the cardiovascular system circulates blood throughout the entire body (macrocirculation), it is the microcirculation (vessel diameter ≤100 µm) that actively and passively regulates erythrocytes and plasma distribution through individual organs and vascular beds.[8]

As early as the nineteenth century, scientists began to conceptualize fluid mechanics and the physical determinants of blood flow. Blood flow is an interplay between the physical principles of hydraulics, pressure, flow, and resistance, whereby the velocity or rate of flow highly depends on the vessel diameter and the characteristics of the fluid (ie, blood viscosity). This relationship can be explained mathematically using Poiseuille's Law[6]:

Flow = Pressure/Resistance

In other words, vascular flow resistance is a function of vascular hindrance (ie, diameter and length) and factors related to blood viscosity. The vascular geometry component of tissue perfusion has been extensively studied in clinical and experimental trials for centuries; however, only within the last 30 years have there been significant advancements in our knowledge and understanding of blood rheology as it relates to tissue perfusion.[2] This dearth in critical knowledge of blood-flow behavior is related to (1) the highly complex nature of the interactions between blood rheologic factors and hemodynamics, and (2) the sensitivity of blood rheologic properties and behaviors to the metabolic status of the surrounding tissue where any tissue-related changes, such as ischemia, make it difficult to determine cause-and-effect relationships in pathophysiologic states.[2] It is well known that the adequacy of blood flow to meet metabolic demands through large circulatory vessels depends highly on vascular control mechanisms. However, the extent to which rheologic properties of blood contributes to vascular flow resistance, particularly in the microcirculation, is less supported by evidence although it is becoming more appreciated.[9] Current evidence suggests that microvascular blood flow is determined by local vessel resistance and hemorheologic factors such as blood viscosity, erythrocyte deformability, and erythrocyte aggregation.[10]

Blood Viscosity

As previously mentioned, blood consists of a cellular component, principally erythrocytes suspended in a relatively homogeneous liquid, the plasma.

Blood viscosity is the flow-determining property of fluid calculated by dividing the shear stress by the shear rate. Viscosity depends on the velocity of flow, temperature, erythrocyte deformability, and the presence of microaggregates. In Newtonian liquids (eg, water) the viscosity is independent of variations in shear stress, so the viscosity remains constant. In non-Newtonian liquids such as blood, viscosity depends on the magnitude of the shear stress or shear rate, and is calculated as a ratio of each.[2] At medium to high shear rates, blood viscosity will increase 4% per unit increase in hematocrit (eg, 45%–46%). For both types of fluids, viscosity is inversely related to the fluid's temperature.

Blood viscosity varies under normal conditions according to the hematocrit ratio (volume of erythrocytes to volume of whole blood)[11] and the diameter of the vessel to which it flows. Plasma, on the other hand, is the suspending element for the cellular components of blood; therefore, any change in plasma viscosity will directly affect blood viscosity regardless of the hematocrit.[2]

As the diameter of the vessel through which blood is traveling progressively becomes smaller, the mean velocity of erythrocytes increases relative to the mean plasma velocity[11] as erythrocytes accumulate and flow in the central zone of the vessel.[2] This characteristic flow behavior of the erythrocytes (central and single-file) leaves plasma to flow peripherally between the erythrocytes and the vessel wall where the shear forces are maximal, resulting in a reduction in viscosity as vessel diameters reach less than 300 μm, approaching a minimum viscosity at diameters of 5 to 7 μm (**Fig. 1**).[12] This reduction in viscosity with reduced vessel diameter is known as the Fåhraeus-Lindqvist effect, whereby the value of blood viscosity is only 10% to 15% greater than that of plasma viscosity in vessels with diameters of 8 to 10 μm.[9] The differences in the mean velocities of the components of blood (ie, erythrocytes and plasma) results in a reduced hematocrit in the microvasculature, often as low as 20%,[13] compared with larger blood vessels (Fåhraeus effect).[14] Lower hematocrit values in the microcirculation relative to systemic hematocrit suggest that oxygen transport to tissues may be compromised as a result of reduced oxygen-carrying capacity.[11] Neither the implications nor the cause-and-effect relationship of reduced microvascular hematocrit values in relation to tissue perfusion are well established.[8]

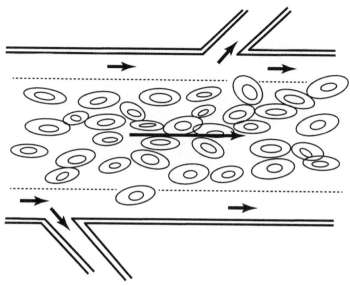

Fig. 1. Accumulation of erythrocytes in the central zone of microvascular blood vessel during flow; vessel periphery (*above and below dotted line*) is the plasma. (*From* Baskurt OK, Meiselman HJ. Blood rheology and hemodynamics. Semin Thromb Hemost 2003;29(5):446; with permission.)

However, studies have shown that erythrocyte deformability plays a significant role in modulating tissue perfusion.[15]

Erythrocyte Deformability

Erythrocytes have a unique biconcave disk shape approximately 8 μm in diameter and 2 μm thick. Behaving as elastic bodies, erythrocytes respond to applied pressure (ie, decrease in vessel diameter) by extensive changes in their shape followed by a reversal when the deforming force is removed. Erythrocyte deformability plays a major role in microvascular tissue perfusion as the oxygen-rich erythrocyte is required to pass through microvessels as small as 3 μm.[6] Erythrocyte-dense blood flowing at progressively greater rates require the erythrocytes to travel in single file separated only by plasma gaps,[12] and become increasingly more deformed, thereby diminishing the viscosity of the blood.[6] This distinct microvascular flow behavior maximizes the surface area available for gas exchange as the erythrocyte transits the capillaries to come into contact with the local tissue environment.[8] Erythrocyte deformability is the most important hemorheologic factor affecting the adequacy of blood flow and tissue perfusion (**Fig. 2**).[3] In pathologic states with reduced erythrocyte deformability (eg, sickle cell disease), erythrocyte sequestering takes place at the capillary entrance, further increasing the resistance to microvascular blood flow.[11,15]

Erythrocyte Aggregation

When suspended in aqueous solutions containing large plasma proteins such as fibrinogen, erythrocytes are able to aggregate to form 2- and 3-dimensional structures. Fibrinogen is the major plasma protein that promotes the formation of erythrocyte aggregation in the blood; there is a linear relationship between fibrinogen concentration and aggregate size.[2] Erythrocytes tend to aggregate into linear

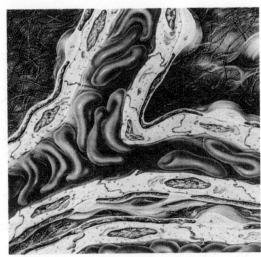

Fig. 2. Erythrocyte deformability. Erythrocytes extensively alter their shape as they flow through the microcirculation. (*From* Baskurt OK, Meiselman HJ. Blood rheology and hemodynamics. Semin Thromb Hemost 2003;29(5):446; with permission.)

arrangements forming an appearance approximating stacked coins (**Fig. 3**). Aggregation depends on the degree of shearing forces acting on the cells where an increased shear environment (ie, high-velocity flow in small microvessels) will discourage aggregation, thus reducing blood viscosity.

Erythrocyte aggregation dominates in conditions of low flow, with increases in viscosity resulting in reduced blood flow in the microcirculation.[9] Alterations in erythrocyte aggregation have been reported in several clinical conditions including sepsis,[16–18] cardiac ischemia and infarction,[19–21] and diabetes mellitus.[22] Further research in the area of microvascular erythrocyte aggregation is needed to fully elucidate its impact on blood flow and tissue oxygenation, as the mechanisms involved in erythrocyte aggregation have not been fully defined.[2] Nevertheless, the hemodynamic consequence of increased erythrocyte aggregation is a decrease in tissue perfusion.

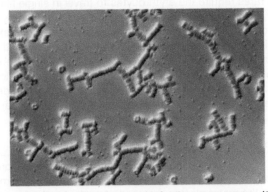

Fig. 3. Erythrocyte aggregates forming stacked-coin appearance. (*From* Baskurt OK, Meiselman HJ. Erythrocyte aggregation: basic aspects and clinical importance. Clin Hemorheol Microcirc. 2013;53(1-2):23–37. Copyright © 2013; with permission from IOS Press.)

ROLE OF LEUKOCYTES IN RESISTANCE

The leukocyte population in blood is very small in comparison with that of erythrocytes; however, leukocytes can generate significant flow resistance on activation in the microcirculation.[23] Leukocytes play a major role in microvascular blood flow because of their flow behavior relative to erythrocytes, which includes stiffness, resistance to deformation, and enhanced viscoelastic characteristics.[1] Consequently, their transit time through the microcirculation is longer and they may even transiently block certain channels.[24] This aspect can be especially concerning in certain pathophysiologic conditions, such as severe infections whereby leukocytes become activated and even more rigid with local occlusive effects. In low-perfusion states (ie, shock), leukocytes can become entrapped in capillaries and may fail to dislodge on return to normal pressure (ie, the no-reflow phenomenon).[5]

SUMMARY

For centuries, researchers have expounded on the knowledge that adequate blood flow to tissues is determined by vascular geometry regulated by vascular control mechanisms in accordance with tissue metabolic demand and viscosity-related factors. Rheologic properties of blood as determinants of vascular flow resistance under dynamic conditions have only recently gained appreciation. Impairments of blood rheologic parameters such as the mechanical properties of erythrocytes and leukocytes will significantly enhance microvascular resistance to blood flow, and may result in impaired perfusion to organs. Knowledge of the behavior of microvascular blood flow promises to be a significant aid to clinicians caring for patients with hemodynamic alterations.

REFERENCES

1. Rampling MW. Compositional properties of blood. In: Baskurt OK, Hardeman MR, Rampling MW, et al, editors. Handbook of hemorheology and hemodynamics. Amsterdam: IOS Press; 2007. p. 34–44.
2. Baskurt OK, Meiselman HJ. Blood rheology and hemodynamics. Semin Thromb Hemost 2003;29(5):435–50.
3. Barvitenko NN, Aslam M, Filosa J, et al. Tissue oxygen demand in regulation of the behavior of the cells in the vasculature. Microcirculation 2013;20(6):484–501.
4. Cooke BM, Lim CT. Mechanical and adhesive properties of healthy and diseased red blood cells. In: Baskurt OK, Hardeman MR, Rampling MW, et al, editors. Handbook of hemorheology and hemodynamics. Amsterdam: IOS; 2007. p. 91–113.
5. Tran-Son-Tay R, Nash GB. Mechanical properties of leukocytes and their effects on the circulation. In: Baskurt OK, Hardeman MR, Rampling MW, et al, editors. Handbook of hemorheology and hemodynamics. Amsterdam: IOS; 2007. p. 137–52.
6. Berne RM, Levy MN. Hemodynamics. In: Cardiovascular physiology. St Louis (MO): Mosby; 2001. p. 115–34.
7. Copley AL. Fluid mechanics and biorheology. Biorheology 1990;27(1):3–19.
8. Bateman RM, Sharpe MD, Ellis CG. Bench-to-bedside review: microvascular dysfunction in sepsis–hemodynamics, oxygen transport, and nitric oxide. Crit Care 2003;7(5):359–73.
9. Meiselman HJ, Baskurt OK. Hemorheology and hemodynamics: dove andare? Clin Hemorheol Microcirc 2006;35(1–2):37–43.

10. Spronk PE, Zandstra DF, Ince C. Bench-to-bedside review: sepsis is a disease of the microcirculation. Crit Care 2004;8(6):462–8.
11. Lipowsky HH. Microvascular rheology and hemodynamics. Microcirculation 2005;12(1):5–15.
12. Pries AR, Secomb TW. Rheology of the microcirculation. Clin Hemorheol Microcirc 2003;29(3–4):143–8.
13. Baskurt OK, Yalcin O, Gungor F, et al. Hemorheological parameters as determinants of myocardial tissue hematocrit values. Clin Hemorheol Microcirc 2006; 35(1–2):45–50.
14. Baskurt OK, Meiselman HJ. Hemodynamic effects of red blood cell aggregation. Indian J Exp Biol 2007;45(1):25–31.
15. Cabrales P. Effects of erythrocyte flexibility on microvascular perfusion and oxygenation during acute anemia. Am J Physiol Heart Circ Physiol 2007;293(2): H1206–15.
16. Alt E, Amann-Vesti BR, Madl C, et al. Platelet aggregation and blood rheology in severe sepsis/septic shock: relation to the sepsis-related organ failure assessment (SOFA) score. Clin Hemorheol Microcirc 2004;30(2):107–15.
17. Berliner AS, Shapira I, Rogowski O, et al. Combined leukocyte and erythrocyte aggregation in the peripheral venous blood during sepsis. An indication of commonly shared adhesive protein(s). Int J Clin Lab Res 2000;30(1):27–31.
18. Kirschenbaum LA, Aziz M, Astiz ME, et al. Influence of rheologic changes and platelet-neutrophil interactions on cell filtration in sepsis. Am J Respir Crit Care Med 2000;161(5):1602–7.
19. Justo D, Mashav N, Arbel Y, et al. Increased erythrocyte aggregation in men with coronary artery disease and erectile dysfunction. Int J Impot Res 2009;21(3): 192–7.
20. Lee BK, Durairaj A, Mehra A, et al. Hemorheological abnormalities in stable angina and acute coronary syndromes. Clin Hemorheol Microcirc 2008;39(1–4): 43–51.
21. Zorio E, Murado J, Arizo D, et al. Haemorheological parameters in young patients with acute myocardial infarction. Clin Hemorheol Microcirc 2008;39(1–4):33–41.
22. Zilberman-Kravits D, Harman-Boehm I, Shuster T, et al. Increased red cell aggregation is correlated with HbA1C and lipid levels in type 1 but not type 2 diabetes. Clin Hemorheol Microcirc 2006;35(4):463–71.
23. Baskurt OK, Meiselman HJ. In vivo hemorheology. In: Baskurt OK, Hardeman MR, Rampling MW, et al, editors. Handbook of hemorheology and hemodynamics. Amsterdam: IOS; 2007. p. 322–38.
24. Eppihimer MJ, Lipowsky HH. Effects of leukocyte-capillary plugging on the resistance to flow in the microvasculature of cremaster muscle for normal and activated leukocytes. Microvasc Res 1996;51(2):187–201.

Monitoring Tissue Blood Flow and Oxygenation
A Brief Review of Emerging Techniques

Penelope S. Benedik, PhD, RN, CRNA, RRT

KEYWORDS

- Physiologic monitoring • Near-infrared spectroscopy • Laser Doppler flowmetry
- Videomicroscopy • Oximetry • Tissue oxygen tension
- Tissue carbon dioxide tension • Lactic acid

KEY POINTS

- Emerging technology should be carefully evaluated prior to implementation and end users should carefully consider the validity of the measurement prior to altering patient therapy.
- Near-infrared spectroscopy, laser Doppler flowmetry, and videomicroscopy may be used to assess perfusion in the microcirculation although each technique has inherent limitations due to their regional nature.
- Tissue oxygen and carbon dioxide levels seem to reflect the extent of tissue metabolism but are also regional in nature.
- Increased lactate levels usually reflect abnormal metabolism but may increase in the absence of cellular hypoxia under certain circumstances.

INTRODUCTION

Understanding the technology that produces physiologic data in terms of its accuracy and precision is an important part of clinical practice. As new technology emerges, it is incumbent on the bedside clinician to understand not only its scientific basis but also the principles of measurement application specific to the new technology. However, technological accuracy and precision will not prevent operator error in the application of devices or the misinterpretation of displayed results. In the clinical setting, operator error is the primary cause of error in measurement.[1]

Measurement issues in clinical practice have been well described. A common example of an operator error is incorrect selection of cuff size or cuff placement during noninvasive oscillometric blood pressure (NIBP) measurement, clearly affecting the accuracy and precision of the measurement value. In addition, NIBP values

Funding Sources: Nil.
Conflict of Interest: Nil.
Division of Nurse Anesthesia, Department of Acute and Continuing Care, University of Texas Health Science Center at Houston, 6901 Bertner, SON 682, Houston, TX 77030, USA
E-mail address: Penelope.s.benedik@uth.tmc.edu

significantly and clinically differ from invasive measures of blood pressure due to patient and disease factors including low systolic pressure, intra- and postoperative instability, atrial fibrillation, or low birth weight.[2–8] Despite the limitations of this ubiquitous technology, NIBP remains a mainstay of patient management in many critical situations. It therefore remains a high priority for bedside clinicians to remain vigilant about the appropriate selection, application, and interpretation of data received from physiologic monitors.

This article describes some of the most promising emerging technologies developed for measuring tissue-level oxygenation or perfusion. Each technique, like all measurement techniques, has its own inherent limitations that should be carefully considered. The end user must understand what the instrument measures and how to interpret the readings. Optical monitoring using near-infrared spectrometry, the Doppler shift, and videomicroscopy are discussed in terms of their application at the tissue level. Assessment of the metabolic state of the extracellular space with existing technology applied in a novel way (oxygen and carbon dioxide electrodes) and proxy indicators of metabolic status (lactate) are discussed. The article also addresses the sources of variation in each measurement and how operator error in the application of these methods can influence patient outcomes.

MEASUREMENT IN CLINICAL PRACTICE

When a novel technology enters the clinical arena, providers are charged with understanding the specifications and limitations of the new instrument. Of particular importance are the accuracy and precision of the device and across what measurement range these specifications apply. The specifications for new technology should be reviewed and evaluated before initiating a new technique in clinical practice (**Box 1**).

Devices used to measure a physiologic variable should meet minimum standards in terms of accuracy and precision, have acceptable sensitivity and specificity, and operate with a clearly defined maximum permissible measurement error.[9]

Box 1
Definitions related to measurement

- *Accuracy* is the closeness of agreement between a measured value and a "true" value
- *Precision* is the closeness of agreement between measured values on the same objects with repeated measurement; also known as measurement reproducibility
- *Sensitivity* communicates the test's ability to identify a positive result; the probability that the test is positive when the patient has the disorder
- *Specificity* communicates a test's ability to identify a negative result; the probability that the test is negative when the patient does not have the disorder
- *Error* is the difference between the measured value and a reference value (used in quality-control procedures)
- *Maximum permissible measurement error* is the extreme value of measurement error, with respect to a known reference value, permitted by specification or regulations for a measuring instrument
- *Calibration error* may occur when a measured value is compared with a known but incorrect standard
- *Offset or zero error* occurs when a device is zeroed against an incorrect value
- *Drift* is a gradual change in the reported measurement when the measured value has not actually changed

Whereas accuracy and precision of a measurement device are generally within a specified range, evaluated and approved by the Food and Drug Administration, and published before entering the market, quality control for the clinical application of the device to the patient is not under rigorous control. For example, there is minimal, if any, training in the proper use and interpretation of automated NIBP data despite its ubiquitous use in acute care settings.[10]

Clinicians must consider whether the novel device is measuring the specific variable of interest or a surrogate variable that is unequivocally associated with the variable of interest. Westgard and Darcy[11] have suggested applying a "truth standard" to the quality of evidence, including clinically measured evidence: the device should measure "all the truth, the whole truth, and nothing but the truth."[11] Applying this concept to the application of new technology, the truth standard might include the following guidelines (adapted from Westgard and Darcy[11]):

- The measurement must have a relationship to the physiologic parameter of interest
- The measurement process must be reliable and provide for correct or "real" test results (eg, instrument accuracy, precision, and application in practice)
- The meaning of the measurement result should not be confounded by other factors (eg, nonspecificity, biological variation of the individual, variation in the interpretation of results)

Both the limits of a new clinical measurement tool and the conditions of measurement should be well defined. For example, a pulse oximeter reading is displayed as a single number, although this number actually represents a range of possible results. The precision of the value displayed depends on the instrument's inherent capability and the proper application of the device. It may be that treatment decisions are based on predefined action values that happen to occur around points of measurement imprecision (see Clinical Box). Clearly, thoughtful and cautious interpretation of physiologic data is an important part of clinical quality control, regardless of the measurement technique.

Clinical Box: Example of technical specifications for pulse oximeter

The accuracy specifications for Nellcor pulse oximeters are usually expressed as "± 2 from 70% to 100% at 1 standard deviation."[a] This means that when the patient's true arterial oxygen saturation falls within the range of 70% to 100%, the Nellcor pulse oximeter will report a saturation that is within 2% of the true saturation about 68% of the time and 4% of the true saturation about 96% of the time.

Therefore 68% of the time, a patient with a reading of 90% could actually have a saturation of 88% to 92%, and 96% of the time a patient with the same reading of 90% has an actual or "true" saturation of 86% to 94%. These ranges clearly intersect possible target values for initiating a change in clinical treatment.

This instrument variation does not account for the within-subject variation that may occur during the measurement (motion artifact[b], weak signal attributable to poor pulse amplitude[c], or venous pulsation[c], to name just a few).

[a] Covidien. Nellcor N-600x pulse oximeter with OxiMax technology. Pamphlet. Boulder (CO): Covidien; 2011.

[b] Petterson MT, Begnoche VL, Graybeal JM. The effect of motion on pulse oximetry and its clinical significance. Anesth Analg 2007;105(Suppl 6):S78–84.

[c] Mannheimer PD. The light-tissue interaction of pulse oximetry. Anesth Analg 2007;105(Suppl 6):S10–7.

Measurement of Tissue Oxygenation

Clinicians historically collect and interpret data on global oxygen delivery and evidence of adequate cellular respiration. Global oxygen delivery (Do_2) is expressed as a product of cardiac output and arterial oxygen content (C_aO_2).

$$Do_2 = \text{Cardiac output} \times C_aO_2$$

$$Do_2 = (\text{Stroke volume} \times \text{heart rate}) \times (\text{Oxygen bound to hemoglobin} + \text{Dissolved oxygen})$$

Although the measurable components of oxygen delivery can be quantified, none of these components directly reflect tissue oxygenation or perfusion. Cardiac output is a measure of ventricular outflow and does not reflect adequate microvascular perfusion, which is under local control.[12] Arterial oxygen content reflects the adequacy of pulmonary gas exchange and oxygen-carrying capacity in the blood but does not reflect the tissue's ability to use oxygen effectively.

The most common clinical methods for quantifying conditions in whole body tissue are indirect measures: mixed venous oxygen saturation and/or lactate levels.[13] These parameters reflect proxy end points of global oxygen consumption and anaerobic metabolism, respectively, and do not reflect regional differences in metabolic activity.[14] Marik has provided a model that frames physiologic data by its relevance to system-level organ failure (**Fig. 1**). Parameters such as cardiac output, blood pressure, and oxygen content represent conditions upstream of the tissue abnormality; they do not reflect tissue-level microcirculation or oxygenation. Mixed venous oxygen levels, base deficit, and lactate are surrogate measures, and only reflect relatively nonspecific global conditions downstream of the tissue lesion.

Techniques that propose to measure evidence of adequate microcirculation and/or local tissue oxygenation are being researched. However, it is important to keep in mind that there is currently no gold standard against which to evaluate the reliability and validity of these techniques. Noninvasive measures of oxygen saturation with pulse oximetry are compared with a purported gold standard of co-oximetry,[15,16] and NIBP values are compared with the gold standard of intra-arterial pressures. At present, no such comparator exists for measures of tissue oxygenation, which may be viewed only as a suggestion about the oxygenation status or perfusion status of the specific tissue bed being monitored.[17] Ekbal and colleagues[14] have categorized new techniques for monitoring regional perfusion by the targeted tissue compartment: the microcirculation, the extracellular space, or the mitochondrion. It is important to bear in mind that these new techniques are neither measures of global oxygen delivery nor proxy values of tissue metabolism; they are regional-level measures of either oxygenation or perfusion at or downstream of the tissue lesion.

Monitors of Perfusion in the Microcirculation

The most promising techniques for measuring tissue perfusion at the level of the microcirculation include near-infrared resonance spectroscopy, laser Doppler flowmetry, and videomicroscopy.

Near-infrared resonance spectroscopy

Optical monitoring is based on the principle that biological media (blood or tissue) absorb, reflect, or scatter light, and that changes in the media alter these optical properties.[18] Optical biosensors have been used clinically for years in the form of pulse oximetry, a technique that uses red and infrared light and a photodetector to measure

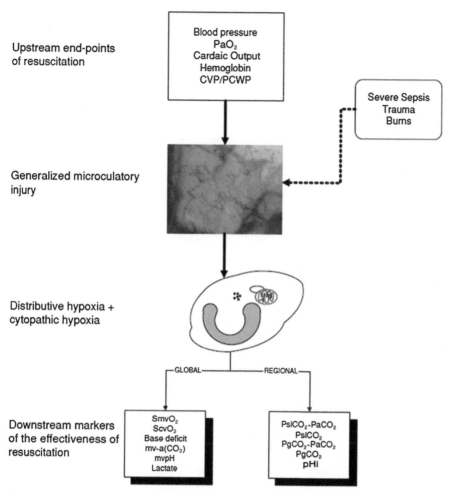

Upstream end-points
of resuscitation

Blood pressure
PaO$_2$
Cardaic Output
Hemoglobin
CVP/PCWP

Severe Sepsis
Trauma
Burns

Generalized microculatory
injury

Distributive hypoxia +
cytopathic hypoxia

—GLOBAL—   —REGIONAL—

Downstream markers
of the effectiveness of
resuscitation

SmvO$_2$
ScvO$_2$
Base deficit
mv-a(CO$_2$)
mvpH
Lactate

PslCO$_2$-PaCO$_2$
PslCO$_2$
PgCO$_2$-PaCO$_2$
PgCO$_2$
pHi

Fig. 1. Conceptual model for evaluating clinical measurement of tissue oxygenation. CVP, central venous pressure; CVWP, central venous wedge pressure; mv-a, mixed venous–arterial; mvpH, mixed venous pH; PaCO$_2$, arterial CO$_2$ partial pressure; PaO$_2$, arterial oxygen partial pressure; PgCO$_2$, gastric intramucosal CO$_2$ partial pressure; pHi, intracellular pH; PslCO$_2$, sublingual CO$_2$ partial pressure; ScvO$_2$, central venous oxygen saturation; SmvO$_2$, mixed venous oxygen saturation. (*From* Marik PE. Sublingual capnometry: a noninvasive measure of microcirculatory dysfunction and tissue hypoxia. Physiol Meas 2006;27(7):R37–47. © Institute of Physics and Engineering in Medicine. Published on behalf of IPEM by IOP Publishing Ltd; p. 39. All rights reserved; with permission.)

the absorbance of oxyhemoglobin and deoxyhemoglobin in a pulsatile tissue bed. Because these 2 wavelengths of light are diminished by bone, muscle, and skin, pulse oximetry targets the pulsatile arterial blood and does not reflect tissue oxygenation.

Near-infrared resonance spectroscopy (NIRS) technology uses infrared and near-infrared light, which reduces the attenuation of the signal by the various tissues.[19] The device measures the change in total hemoglobin and oxygenated hemoglobin, which represents the tissue oxygenation saturation (Sto$_2$) for the tissue bed in question. As such, NIRS is considered a tissue-specific assessment of oxygen

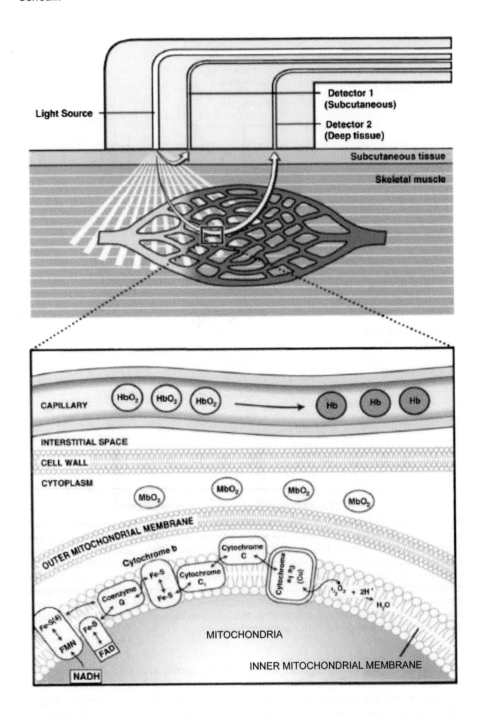

availability.[20] NIRS technology allows for the contribution of oxygen bound to myoglobin and mitochondrial cytochrome oxidase to StO_2, although their contribution is minor (**Fig. 2**).

NIRS technology has been used for the assessment of cerebral oxygenation using emitters and detectors placed on the forehead to measure regional cortical oxygenation (rSO_2) in neonates and during cerebral and vascular surgery.[21] The NIRS value is assumed to represent oxygenation in the brain tissue approximately 2.5 cm below the surface of the scalp.[22] To measure peripheral tissue oxygenation, the device is generally placed on the thenar eminence, a superficial muscle on the palmar surface of the hand. Because most blood distribution in muscle is venous, NIRS StO_2 likely represents local venous oxygen saturation rather than tissue values.[14]

NIRS readings have been reported to precede changes in base deficit, lactate levels, and hemodynamics, suggesting that it may serve as an early indicator of organ ischemia. Of note, StO_2 may also reflect changes in blood flow and/or local metabolism, confounding its interpretation in septic patients or those in traumatic shock. StO_2 has been shown to be an independent predictor of the need for massive transfusion, and persistently low StO_2 values predict poor outcomes in animal models and human studies.[19,23]

NIRS values are affected by adipose tissue thickness, edema, hypoalbuminemia, endothelial leak syndromes, venous congestion, age, body mass index, sex, race, and ethnicity.[14,24] The thenar eminence is the site of choice for peripheral monitoring, as it has a relatively thin fat layer, accumulates less edema, and exhibits less pigmentation than other accessible peripheral sites.[21] Alternative sites that have been suggested include the forearm, pectoral muscle, or deltoid muscle. A major limitation of NIRS when applied to a peripheral muscle bed is the lack of differentiation between myoglobin and hemoglobin saturation. In this setting, oxyhemoglobin values may be overestimated. These user-dependent choices will likely affect the clinical validity and reliability of NIRS data. Although trends in StO_2 may not adequately represent trends in central venous oxygen saturation,[25] NIRS is commonly used to trend regional cerebral oxygenation during vascular surgery, and is associated with improved patient outcomes.[26]

Laser Doppler flowmetry

Laser Doppler flowmetry (LDF) is another optical technology that provides information about blood flow to a tissue bed using visible and infrared light. The Doppler shift that

---

Fig. 2. Near-infrared spectroscopy (NIRS) in the reflectance mode overlying skin and skeletal muscle. NIRS is capable of providing information concerning the balance between oxygen delivery and consumption of an organ(s) by assessing the state of hemoglobin oxygen saturation (HbO_2) in the microvasculature and intracellular oxygen utilization via the redox state of cytochrome oxidase. The value and measure of tissue oxygen saturation (StO_2) lies in the distribution of blood in the organ of interest, with approximately 70% of blood volume being in the venous compartment under normal conditions. When NIRS is used to assess skeletal muscle perfusion, the contribution of myoglobin must be taken into account. Note that the technology illustrated here might allow differentiation of the NIRS radiation returning from the subcutaneous tissue from deeper underlying tissues such as skeletal muscle. Because light follows an elliptical pathway, spacing of detectors at various distances from the light source assist in determining the origin of the returning signal. FAD, flavin adenine dinucleotide; FMN, flavin mononucleotide; MbO_2, oxymyoglobin; NADH, reduced nicotinamide adenine dinucleotide. (*From* Ward KR, Ivatury RR, Barbee RW, et al. Near infrared spectroscopy for evaluation of the trauma patient: a technology review. Resuscitation 2006;68:31; with permission.)

occurs when light encounters moving erythrocytes is detected, and is proportional to perfusion in the detectable field (0.5–1 mm^3).[14,17] Because the depth of laser penetration is low, measurement is limited to skin or mucous membranes. LDF has been closely correlated with other measures of blood-flow measurement techniques, and is an assessment of tissue perfusion, not oxygenation.[20]

Like NIRS, laser technology may demonstrate earlier changes when compared with base deficit, lactate, heart rate, and blood pressure change in traumatic shock conditions. LDF is quantified in arbitrary units, not absolute blood flow; therefore, the provider can only use it for trending. Its accuracy is reduced in tissue beds with heterogeneous blood flow because the Doppler senses multiple vessels with flow moving in different directions within the field. Moving the Doppler probe to obtain values will alter the ability to trend flow, so the probe should be fixed into position.

Videomicroscopic techniques

Microscopic examination of skin or mucosal surfaces provides an image of local perfusion, that is, a direct visualization of blood in the microcirculation, and has been used in tissue beds with thin epithelial layers (sublingual, brain, intestine, liver).[27] The microscopic field generally includes capillaries and venules, but may exclude arterioles because of their anatomically deeper position in the tissue bed.[17] The sidestream dark-field imaging technique allows erythrocytes to be visualized as black bodies moving across a white background, revealing the flow of blood in individual vessels (**Fig. 3**).[14]

The intensity of illumination and the depth of focus must be adjusted to ensure an adequate visual quality of the imaged structures. Images are not reviewed in real time; recorded images are subjected to both manual and software analyses that are semiquantitative in nature.[14] The examination of a stored visual image includes an assessment of capillary density (identifying and counting the capillaries within a specific area) and examining the structural characteristics of the capillary bed.[27] Thus videomicroscopy is time consuming, requires significant training, and provides only an intermittent assessment of a portion of the selected microcirculatory vasculature.

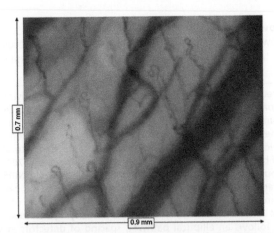

Fig. 3. Videomicroscopic image of labial microvasculature using sidestream dark-field imaging. Capillaries are loops emerging from the shadowy arterioles visualized in the background. (*From* Djaberi R, Schuijf JD, de Koning EJ, et al. Non-invasive assessment of microcirculation by sidestream dark field imaging as a marker of coronary artery disease in diabetes. Diab Vasc Dis Res 2013;10(2):125; with permission.)

Altered sublingual microcirculation has been demonstrated in septic and cardiogenic shock and, in a few limited studies, pharmacologic intervention improved microcirculation. However, therapy that improved microcirculatory flow did not alter overall morbidity or mortality.

Monitors of the Extracellular Environment

The metabolic state of local tissue may be reflected by the tissue oxygen level, tissue carbon dioxide level, or the accumulation of metabolic by-products (eg, lactate, pyruvate, glycerol). These measurements may be either direct or indirect indicators of tissue health.

Tissue oxygen tension

The partial pressure of dissolved oxygen has traditionally been measured with the Clark electrode, the technology used to measure the partial pressure of dissolved oxygen (Po_2) in a blood gas analyzer. In this classic polarographic technique, oxygen diffuses across the electrode membrane and is reduced at a rate proportional to the tissue Po_2 (tPo_2). However, this method consumes oxygen, which may decrease its accuracy at the low tPo_2 levels in various organ beds. Polarographic electrodes embedded in the brain parenchyma have been used effectively to guide therapy in patents with cerebral injury.[28] The reported tPo_2 is highly accurate and precise, but the data are limited by the probe measuring only the tissue bed within 7 to 15 mm^2 of the probe tip (about 1/50th to 1/100th of a square inch). In addition, probe location in the brain will critically affect the measured value of tPo_2: values in injured brain will differ markedly from those in uninjured brain. Brain tPo_2 notably supplies no information about the metabolic state of the cerebral tissue, although management of traumatic brain injury using polarographically derived tPo_2 has resulted in small improvements in outcome.

Photoluminescence quenching is a technique that couples a transfer of energy to oxygen from a light-excited luminophore within a tiny fiberoptic cable. The resulting luminescence decays at a rate inversely proportional to the tPo_2; because no oxygen is consumed, the technique is fitting in a low oxygen environment.[14,29] Sensors can be precalibrated and are being developed for patient use.

Tissue carbon dioxide

Carbon dioxide is produced by tissue metabolism and removed by local tissue perfusion; tissue CO_2, however, is determined by arterial CO_2, regional perfusion, and tissue CO_2 (tco_2) production. An increase in tco_2 most likely represents a decrease in local tissue blood flow because increases in CO_2 production are associated with parallel increases in vasodilation that keep tco_2 constant.[30] Often the clinician will follow the tissue to arterial CO_2 gradient, or CO_2 gap, which reflects that adequacy of tissue perfusion.[17] Conditions associated with poor tissue perfusion are highly associated with increases in gastric tco_2 as measured by both gastric tonometry and sublingual capnometry.[14]

Whereas gastric tonometry is relatively invasive and difficult to perform, placement of a disposable CO_2 sensor under the tongue is highly feasible. The technology is based on a luminescence technique in which CO_2 diffuses across the sensor membrane, dissociates into hydrogen ions, which alters pH, and modifies the fluorescent properties of a pH-sensitive dye. The device measures sublingual partial pressure of CO_2 ($Pslco_2$), and provides a resolution of 0.1 mm Hg at CO_2 levels less than 70 mm Hg and 0.3 mm Hg when CO_2 levels exceed 150 mm Hg.[31] The tongue and sublingual mucosa appear to adequately perform as an extension of the relatively sensitive splanchnic circulation in this regard.

Lactate

Lactate has been proposed as an estimate of disease severity and to monitor disease course, because of its link to tissue hypoxia. A thorough review of lactate monitoring was recently published that supports the use of lactate trending in resuscitation protocols despite its lack of specificity as a global marker of tissue oxygenation.[32]

Under normal or aerobic conditions in healthy tissue, glucose is metabolized in the glycolytic pathway to pyruvate, which typically enters the Krebs cycle for further oxidation in the mitochondria. In anaerobic conditions, oxidative phosphorylation is inhibited and pyruvate is diverted to lactate. When cellular recovery occurs and oxygen is available, the mitochondria proceed with the Krebs cycle and the remaining lactate is converted back to pyruvate (**Fig. 4**). Conversion of pyruvate to lactate allows the glycolytic pathway to proceed unhampered by the negative feedback of its accumulated substrate. Thus a cell's ability to consume oxygen may be indicated by the shunting of pyruvate to lactate rather than proceeding into the Krebs cycle and oxidative phosphorylation.

Lactate levels higher than 5.0 mmol/L are only weakly associated with arterial pH of less than 7.35; lactate levels lower than 5.0 mmol/L are poorly correlated with pH. Lactate-associated metabolic acidosis has a higher risk of mortality than other causes of metabolic acidosis. When oxygen consumption exceeds oxygen delivery, dramatic increases in lactate are observed; however, once aerobic metabolism resumes, lactate is rapidly cleared.

A conundrum occurs in the clinical interpretation of lactate because several conditions increase lactate even in the absence of cellular hypoxia. Increases in aerobic glucose metabolism produced by epinephrine administration cause dose-dependent increases in lactate; patients who require catecholamine infusions are likely suffering from impaired tissue perfusion. Both metabolic and respiratory alkalosis stimulate phosphofructokinase, a key enzyme in the glycolytic pathway, and this process increases lactate levels independent of oxygen status. Metformin use and propofol administration have also been associated with increased lactate. Lactate may accumulate when its clearance is decreased, and this has been demonstrated in liver dysfunction and sepsis. In critically ill septic patients, lactate clearance was an independent predictor of outcome.[33]

Although lactate levels usually reflect abnormal oxidative metabolism, it is clearly important that the clinician evaluate all of the potential causes of hyperlactatemia.

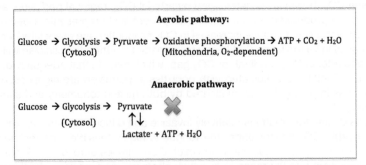

Aerobic pathway:

Glucose → Glycolysis → Pyruvate → Oxidative phosphorylation → $ATP + CO_2 + H_2O$
(Cytosol) (Mitochondria, O_2-dependent)

Anaerobic pathway:

Glucose → Glycolysis → Pyruvate
(Cytosol)   ↑↓
Lactate⁻ + ATP + H_2O

Fig. 4. Glycolytic pathway. Under normal or aerobic conditions in healthy tissue, glucose is metabolized in the glycolytic pathway to pyruvate, which typically enters the Krebs cycle for further oxidation in the mitochondria. Under anaerobic conditions, oxidative phosphorylation is inhibited and pyruvate is diverted to lactate. When cellular recovery occurs and oxygen is available, the mitochondria proceed with the Krebs cycle and the remaining lactate is converted back to pyruvate.

Sampling sites and devices should be consistent when trending lactate levels so as to avoid the inevitable instrument variability.

SUMMARY

Many of the newest techniques for assessing tissue oxygenation and/or perfusion cannot yet pass the major points in the truth standard. The downstream measures, tissue Po_2 and tissue Pco_2, partially satisfy the first requirement: they have a clear relationship to the measurement of interest. However, the meaning of these data may be confounded by a variety of other factors because they only reflect regional conditions. Using lactate levels as a global measure of tissue metabolism has well-described limitations. Promising monitors of tissue blood flow (NIRS, laser Doppler, and videomicroscopy) are limited by their regional nature, technical difficulty in application, and data that are confounded by both biological and interpretive variation.

As these new technologies enter the critical care arena, key components of their utility will be the appropriate application of the devices and the proper calibration before and during use by the end user; in other words, quality control cannot stop at the level of the manufacturer. The end user must understand what the instrument is intended to measure, and the interpretation of the measurement must be thoughtfully considered before the data are used to alter patient therapy.

REFERENCES

1. Byrne A. Error in clinical measurement. Anaesthesia and Intensive Care Medicine 2011;12(12):578–80.
2. Lehman LW, Saeed M, Talmor D, et al. Methods of blood pressure measurement in the ICU. Crit Care Med 2013;41(1):34–40.
3. Lakhal K, Macq C, Ehrmann S, et al. Noninvasive monitoring of blood pressure in the critically ill: reliability according to the cuff site (arm, thigh, or ankle). Crit Care Med 2012;40(4):1207–13.
4. Tao G, Chen Y, Wen C, et al. Statistical analysis of blood pressure measurement errors by oscillometry during surgical operations. Blood Press Monit 2011;16(6): 285–90.
5. Chatterjee A, DePriest K, Blair R, et al. Results of a survey of blood pressure monitoring by intensivists in critically ill patients: a preliminary study. Crit Care Med 2010;38(12):2335–8.
6. Troy R, Doron M, Laughon M, et al. Comparison of noninvasive and central arterial blood pressure measurements in ELBW infants. J Perinatol 2009;29(11):744–9.
7. Anastas ZM, Jimerson E, Garolis S. Comparison of noninvasive blood pressure measurements in patients with atrial fibrillation. J Cardiovasc Nurs 2008;23(6): 519–24 [quiz: 525–6].
8. Smulyan H, Safar ME. Blood pressure measurement: retrospective and prospective views. Am J Hypertens 2011;24(6):628–34.
9. Joint Committee for Guides in Metrology (JCGM). International vocabulary of metrology—basic and general concepts and associated terms. 2012 (E/F).
10. de Greeff A, Shennan A. Blood pressure measuring devices: ubiquitous, essential but imprecise. Expert Rev Med Devices 2008;5(5):573–9.
11. Westgard JO, Darcy T. The truth about quality: medical usefulness and analytical reliability of laboratory tests. Clin Chim Acta 2004;346(1):3–11.
12. Spiess B. Critical oxygen delivery, the microcirculation and cardiac surgery: what we know now and need to know! J of Extra Corpor Technol 2011;43(1):10–6.

13. Tanczos K, Molnar Z. The oxygen supply-demand balance: a monitoring challenge. Best Pract Res Clin Anaesthesiol 2013;27(2):201–7.
14. Ekbal NJ, Dyson A, Black C, et al. Monitoring tissue perfusion, oxygenation, and metabolism in critically ill patients. Chest 2013;143(6):1799–808.
15. Zaouter C, Zavorsky GS. The measurement of carboxyhemoglobin and methemoglobin using a non-invasive pulse CO-oximeter. Respir Physiol Neurobiol 2012;182(2–3):88–92.
16. Gehring H, Duembgen L, Peterlein M, et al. Hemoximetry as the "gold standard"? Error assessment based on differences among identical blood gas analyzer devices of five manufacturers. Anesth Analg 2007;105(Suppl 6):S24–30.
17. De Backer D, Donadello K, Cortes DO. Monitoring the microcirculation. J Clin Monit Comput 2012;26(5):361–6.
18. Mendelson Y. Biomedical sensors. In: Enderle J, Blanchard S, Bronzino J, editors. Introduction to biomedical engineering. 2nd edition. Burlington (MA): Elsevier; 2005. p. 505–48.
19. Hampton DA, Schreiber MA. Near infrared spectroscopy: clinical and research uses. Transfusion 2013;53(Suppl 1):52S–8S.
20. Sakr Y. Techniques to assess tissue oxygenation in the clinical setting. Transfus Apher Sci 2010;43(1):79–94.
21. Scheeren TW, Schober P, Schwarte LA. Monitoring tissue oxygenation by near infrared spectroscopy (NIRS): background and current applications. J Clin Monit Comput 2012;26(4):279–87.
22. Pattison K, Wynne-Jones G, Imray C. Monitoring intracranial pressure, perfusion and metabolism. Cont Educ Anaesth Crit Care Pain 2005;5(4):130–3.
23. Moore FA, Nelson T, McKinley BA, et al. Massive transfusion in trauma patients: tissue hemoglobin oxygen saturation predicts poor outcome. J Trauma 2008;64(4):1010–23.
24. Wolf U, Wolf M, Choi JH, et al. Mapping of hemodynamics of the human calf with near infrared spectroscopy and the influence of the adipose tissue thickness. In: Wilson DF, Evans SM, Giaglow J, Pastuszko A, editors. Oxygen transport to tissue XXIII. Vol. 510. Philadelphia: Kluwer Acedemic/Plenum 2003;203:225–30.
25. Fellahi JL, Fischer MO, Rebet O, et al. Cerebral and somatic near-infrared spectroscopy measurements during fluid challenge in cardiac surgery patients: a descriptive pilot study. J Cardiothorac Vasc Anesth 2013;27(2):266–72.
26. Murkin JM, Arango M. Near-infrared spectroscopy as an index of brain and tissue oxygenation. Br J Anaesth 2009;103(Suppl 1):i3–13.
27. Djaberi R, Schuijf JD, de Koning EJ, et al. Non-invasive assessment of microcirculation by sidestream dark field imaging as a marker of coronary artery disease in diabetes. Diab Vasc Dis Res 2013;10(2):123–34.
28. Martini RP, Deem S, Treggiari MM. Targeting brain tissue oxygenation in traumatic brain injury. Respir Care 2013;58(1):162–72.
29. Dmitriev RI, Papkovsky DB. Optical probes and techniques for O_2 measurement in live cells and tissue. Cell Mol Life Sci 2012;69(12):2025–39.
30. Marik PE. Regional carbon dioxide monitoring to assess the adequacy of tissue perfusion. Curr Opin Crit Care 2005;11(3):245–51.
31. Marik PE. Sublingual capnometry: a non-invasive measure of microcirculatory dysfunction and tissue hypoxia. Physiol Meas 2006;27(7):R37–47.
32. Bakker J, Nijsten MW, Jansen TC. Clinical use of lactate monitoring in critically ill patients. Ann Intensive Care 2013;3(1):12.
33. Nguyen HB, Kuan WS, Batech M, et al. Outcome effectiveness of the severe sepsis resuscitation bundle with addition of lactate clearance as a bundle item: a multi-national evaluation. Crit Care 2011;15(5):R229.

Exploring Hemodynamics
A Review of Current and Emerging
Noninvasive Monitoring Techniques

 CrossMark

Alexander Johnson, MSN, RN, ACNP-BC, CCNS, CCRN*,
Mehr Mohajer-Esfahani, BSN, RN

KEYWORDS

• Stroke volume • Hemodynamics • Cardiac output • Hypovolemia

KEY POINTS

• The lack of randomized controlled trials suggesting improved outcomes with pulmonary artery catheter use and pressure-based hemodynamic monitoring has led to a decrease in pulmonary artery catheter use.
• An increasing amount of literature supporting stroke volume optimization (SVO) has given rise to a paradigm shift from pressure-based to flow-based techniques.
• Regardless of the device chosen, the SVO algorithm approach should be considered, and volume challenges should be guided by dynamic assessments of fluid responsiveness. Although SVO requires further study in extubated and medical intensive care unit populations, a mortality benefit has been observed in high-risk surgical patients.
• The use of SVO is supported by more evidence than for central venous pressure for fluid resuscitation.

INTRODUCTION

Over the last 15 years, hemodynamic monitoring has evolved. Monitoring technologies and resuscitation strategies are transitioning from pressure-based parameters (such as central venous pressure [CVP]) to flow-based parameters (such as cardiac output and stroke volume [SV]) as the supporting evidence increases for a protocolized approach to hemodynamic optimization rather than traditional approaches. Early goal-directed therapy protocols are an emerging standard of practice that is no longer limited to the care of patients with sepsis. This article provides a general overview of the paradigm shift occurring in hemodynamic monitoring, including current monitoring techniques, resuscitation end points, and supporting evidence. In contrast with many other hemodynamic review articles, this article also focuses on practical application

Conflict of Interest: None.
Critical Care, Central DuPage Hospital, Cadence Health, 25 North Winfield Road, Winfield, IL 60190, USA
* Corresponding author.
E-mail address: apjccrn@hotmail.com

and systematic use of technology so that cardiac output and SV can be optimized regardless of the device used.

Before deliberating over the emerging trends and latest devices in hemodynamic monitoring, it is worthwhile to discuss the goals of monitoring and hemodynamic optimization. The goals of this concept are largely concerned with 2 objectives: (1) optimizing the macrocirculation (eg, cardiac output, SV), and (2) optimizing the tissue oxygenation via end points such as blood lactate, central venous oxygen saturation ($ScvO_2$), and mixed venous oxygen saturation (SvO_2) levels. This article discusses the macrocirculatory parameters of hemodynamic optimization as they relate to current and emerging trends in hemodynamic monitoring.

FROM CARDIAC PRESSURES TO PARAMETERS BASED ON BLOOD FLOW

In the past, cardiac filling pressures were associated with a proportionate cardiac filling volume. However, recent studies suggest that cardiac pressures do not consistently correlate with cardiac volume. A systematic review of the literature was published in *Chest* in 2008 by Marik and colleagues.[1] That study examined every article published to date on the ability of the CVP to predict preload responsiveness or cardiac output after a fluid challenge in humans (24 studies met the inclusion criteria, n = 803). In that review, Marik and colleagues[1] could find no data to suggest that the CVP correlated well with intravascular volume status or preload. The investigators thus concluded that the CVP should no longer be used to make clinical decisions regarding fluid management. The pooled correlation coefficient between CVP and measured blood volume was 0.16 (95% confidence interval, 0.03–0.28), which suggests that the accuracy of CVP for measuring blood volume is like flipping a coin.[1] Similar studies have been published regarding the poor correlation between the pulmonary artery occlusive pressure (PAOP) and left ventricular end-diastolic volume.[2–5] Several clinical factors can exacerbate this poor correlation between pressure and volume (ie, factors that alter the pressure-compliance curve of the myocardium). These factors include mechanical ventilation, aging, obesity, history of myocardial infarction, diabetes, and sepsis.[6] The primary reason to administer a fluid challenge is to increase the SV (or cardiac output), not static cardiac filling pressures such as PAOP or CVP. The PAOP and CVP were intended to be guides to better optimize cardiac output and SV.

Meanwhile, the last 10 years have produced other studies that have highlighted the slow-to-change and misleading nature of other commonly used monitoring parameters in critical care. In 1996, Hamilton-Davies and colleagues[7] published an observational study that showed the limitations of traditional vital signs as early indicators of volume depletion. Six healthy volunteers were phlebotomized of a mean 25.3% (standard deviation [SD], 3.5%) of their respective blood volumes over 90 minutes. Systolic blood pressure, heart rate, and SV were among the parameters continuously monitored. After the 90-minute target time, the only statistically significant change in these parameters was in the SV. Average SV decreased by a mean of 16.5 mL (SD, 15 mL; $P<.01$). Systolic blood pressure and heart rate failed to show consistent or significant changes (**Fig. 1**). These findings suggest that pressure-based parameters and traditional vital signs may not equate to blood flow–based parameters, and that flow decreases before pressure decreases as hypovolemia worsens.

USE OF SV TO ASSESS FLUID RESPONSIVENESS
SV Optimization

The study by Hamilton-Davies and colleagues[7] suggests a temporal order of events in hypovolemia, beginning with a decrease in SV when a decrease in overall circulating

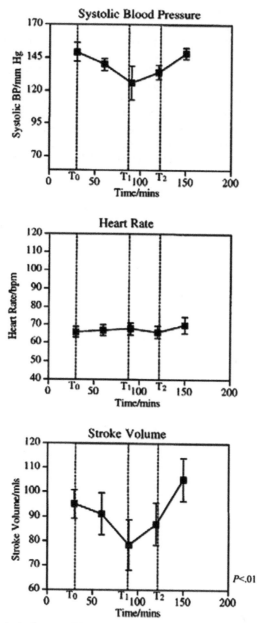

Fig. 1. SV as an early indicator of hypovolemia compared with traditional vital signs. The progressive hemodynamic response to volume depletion in healthy volunteers. T_0 is baseline, T_1 is end of bleed, T_2 is before retransfusion. The P value is the significance at end of bleed relative to baseline. The decrease in SV was statistically significant, whereas heart rate and systolic blood pressure remained essentially unchanged. (*From* Hamilton-Davies C, Mythen M, Salmon J, et al. Comparison of commonly used clinical indicators of hypovolaemia with gastrointestinal tonometry. Intensive Care Med 1997;23(3):279; with permission.)

volume is the precipitating event. The study suggests that all other physiologic changes caused by hypovolemia, including tachycardia, low urine output, and altered mental status, are compensatory responses to the change in SV. The Advanced Trauma Life Support Hemorrhagic Classification Scale[8] also suggests a characteristic sequence of events in hypovolemia. This scale displays characteristic ranges for monitoring parameters in 4 classes, ranging from class 1 (<15% blood loss) to class 4 (>40% blood loss). Blood pressure is not shown to decrease until class 3 (30%–40% blood loss), which further suggests that flow-related parameters may be earlier indicators of hypovolemia than pressure-related parameters.[8]

This sequence of events, preceded by a decrease in SV, has led to a new targeted resuscitation strategy termed SV optimization (SVO). **Fig. 2** shows a conventional SVO

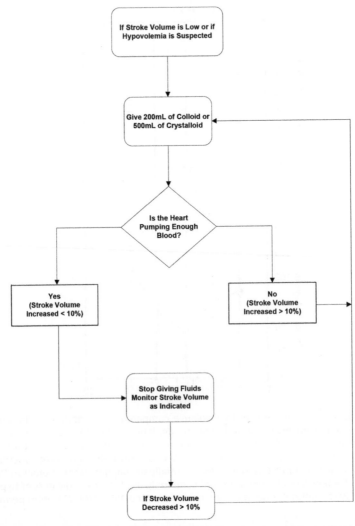

Fig. 2. Typical SVO algorithm based on a synthesis of protocols used in randomized trials.

resuscitation algorithm. The algorithm is predicated on the concept that fluid responsiveness (ie, recruitable cardiac output) is determined by an increase in SV of 10% or more after a fluid challenge. The algorithm guides the clinician to continue fluid challenges as long as the SV continues to improve by at least 10% (a dynamic marker of fluid responsiveness). When SV ceases to improve by at least 10%, this indicates that the point of diminishing returns, or the plateaued portion along the Starling curve, is achieved and the algorithm directs the clinician to stop giving volume challenges (**Fig. 3**). This algorithm has been used as a clinical protocol and was studied with replication in 9 randomized controlled trials (RCTs) in the perioperative population. Those trials consistently reported patient benefits, such as decreased intensive care unit (ICU) length of stay, decreased hospital length of stay, decreased blood lactate levels, decreased vasopressor use, improved time to tolerating oral intake, and decreased complication rates compared with controls (**Table 1**).[9–17] A systematic review of the literature conducted by the National Health Service (NHS), which included 8 of these randomized trials (n = 959) as well as others, further validated that SVO consistently contributes to decreased postoperative morbidity and length of stay.[18]

Passive Leg Raise Maneuver

Another highly predictive and dynamic method of assessing fluid responsiveness is with the passive leg raise (PLR) maneuver.[19] With the patient beginning in a recumbent 30° to 45° supine position, lowering the trunk to the flat position and elevating the legs to 45° autotransfuses the patient and allows the clinician to assess for a fluid challenge response without administering exogenous intravenous fluid. In a recent study performed in a medical ICU using noninvasive Doppler, Thiel and colleagues[20] found

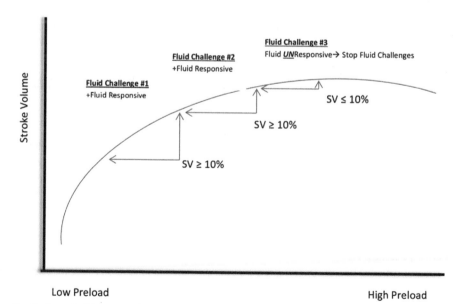

Fig. 3. Recruitable SV; Starling curve. SV improves by 10% or more with successive fluid challenges, which suggests that the patient is preload responsive. The steep portion of the curve represents an area of recruitable cardiac output. The flat portion represents a euvolemic state.

Table 1
RCTs using the esophageal Doppler

Reference, Year	Perioperative Patient Population	n	Primary Outcomes (SVO Group vs Conventional Care)
Mythen & Webb,[13] 1995	Cardiac surgery	60	↓ Complications in SVO group (0 vs 6, $P = .01$) ↓ LOS (6.4 vs 10.1 d, $P = .023$) in SVO
Sinclair et al,[14] 1997	Proximal femoral fracture surgery	40	↓ LOS (10 vs 18 d)
Gan et al,[11] 2002	General, urologic, or gynecologic surgery	98	↓ LOS (5 vs 7 d [mean], $P = .03$) ↓ Severe postoperative N/v in SVO ($P = .01$)
Venn et al,[15] 2002	Proximal femoral fracture surgery	90	↓ Time medical fit for discharge (by 6.2 d) in SVO group
Conway et al,[10] 2002	Major bowel surgery	57	↑ ICU admissions in conventional care group (0 in SVO group vs 5 in control)
McKendry et al,[12] 2004	Cardiac critical care unit (postoperative)	174	↓ Mean ICU days (2.5 in SVO from 3.2) ↓ LOS (11.4 vs 13.9 d)
Wakeling et al,[16] 2005	Major bowel surgery	128	↓ LOS (median) (10 vs 11 d, $P = .05$)
Noblett et al,[17] 2006	Colorectal resection	103	↓ LOS (7 vs 9 d, $P = .005$) ↓ Time to tolerate oral intake (by 2 d, $P = .029$) ↓ Morbidity in SVO group (1 vs 8, $P = .043$)
Chytra et al,[9] 2007	Patients with trauma in critical care unit	162	↓ Lactate levels (2.92 mmol/L vs 3.22 mmol/L, $P = .003$) ↓ LOS (14 vs 17.5 d, median, $P = .045$) ↓ ICU LOS (7 vs 8.5 d, $P = .031$)

Abbreviations: LOS, length of stay; N/v, nausea and vomiting.

that an SV increase of greater than or equal to 15% induced by PLR predicted volume responsiveness with a sensitivity of 81%, specificity of 93%, positive predictive value of 91%, and negative predictive value of 85%. Monnet and colleagues[21] found slightly better predictability in a similarly designed study using esophageal Doppler (97% sensitivity, 94% specificity). The investigators reported improvements in cardiac output in response to PLR in less than 1 minute.

TECHNIQUES FOR ASSESSING SV AT THE BEDSIDE

The echocardiogram is currently the gold standard for measuring SV at the bedside. Although the echocardiogram is highly accurate, it is expensive, requires a specially trained technician, and is less conducive to ongoing serial measurements in critical care. The remainder of this article reviews the alternative methods of the pulmonary artery catheter (PAC), Doppler techniques, pulse contour techniques, bioimpedance, and bioreactance.

PAC

In 1996, Connors and colleagues[22] published a prospective, multicenter cohort study (n = 5735) in critically ill patients that suggested that PACs are associated with an increase in mortality. Since then, practice trends in hemodynamic monitoring have shown a general decrease in PAC use as clinicians began searching for a minimally invasive alternative. Subsequent systematic reviews suggesting no benefit for PAC use performed by the Agency for Healthcare Research and Quality (AHRQ)[23] and the Cochrane Collaboration[24] indicate that this trend in decreased PAC use is likely to continue. The AHRQ and Cochrane Collaboration cite many factors why PAC studies suggest a lack of patient benefit. Among them, inconsistent use and lack of protocolized use are fundamental reasons,[23,24] which is in contrast with the SVO protocol used in each of the 9 RCTs studying SVO.[9–17] The data published by Connors and colleagues[22] may suggest that it may not be the PAC that has contributed to a perceived lack of benefit, but perhaps the clinicians who used PACs in the studies meeting the inclusion criteria.

Doppler Techniques

The 9 RCTs mentioned earlier that studied the SVO treatment algorithm were all performed by using the esophageal Doppler. The existence of so many trials is partially the result of ultrasonography applications such as the esophageal Doppler for ongoing cardiac output monitoring at the bedside having been established since the 1970s.

Description

The Doppler principle is well known and validated across multiple professions, from engineering to medicine. An ultrasound beam is emitted from the transducer and reflects off red blood cells passing by the beam path. Ultrasound waves reflected back toward the transducer provide information regarding the speed, acceleration, velocity, and distance a column of blood travels during the cardiac cycle. The monitor uses the information from the ultrasound waves to produce hemodynamic values.

Techniques

The esophageal Doppler (Deltex Medical, United Kingdom) is the technique with the most research to support its use in SVO (Fig. 4). In this technique, a 14-French ultrasound probe is inserted into the patient's esophagus to a depth of approximately 30 to 40 cm (about T5–T6 level). The probe is then twisted slightly until the ultrasound beam is directed at the descending thoracic aorta, which creates an aortic pulse wave on the monitor (Fig. 5).

The second most common ultrasonography method for hemodynamic monitoring is the external (noninvasive) Doppler (USCOM, Sydney, Australia). This technique uses ultrasound to obtain values similar to the esophageal Doppler hemodynamic values; however, the external Doppler does this less invasively. The clinician places the ultrasound probe at the sternal notch and angles the beam at the aortic valve, or places the probe parasternally, angling the beam at the pulmonic valve.

Advantages

The minimally invasive applications, ease of use, and accuracy are advantages of the Doppler methods. Neither the esophageal Doppler nor the external Doppler requires any invasive lines. The transcutaneous application of the external Doppler allows it to be used in outpatient settings and clinics. Although the Doppler methods are easy to use, use of the esophageal Doppler is easier to learn. Clinicians typically develop competency with signal acquisition after approximately 3 esophageal Doppler insertions. However, the noninvasive Doppler typically requires approximately 20 attempts for users to achieve competency.

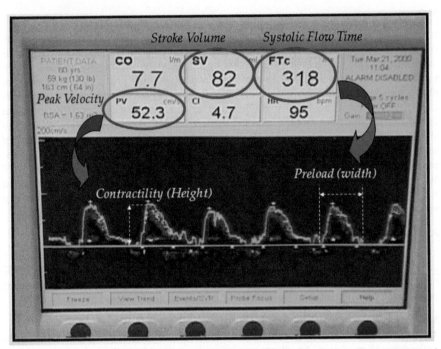

Fig. 4. Esophageal Doppler patient monitor. Most minimally invasive cardiac output monitors produce metrics for preload, afterload, and contractility in order to optimize SV (normal = 50–120 mL). For example, on this typical esophageal Doppler monitor, (1) preload is indicated by FTc (systolic flow time; normal = 330–360 milliseconds), which represents the time spent in systole, corrected for heart rate. FTc often corresponds with the width of the aortic pulse wave. (2) Contractility is measured by the peak velocity (PV; normal = 50–100 cm/s), which often corresponds to the amplitude of the wave. (3) SVR can also be calculated and displayed on a different screen, although SVR is generally considered a secondary monitoring parameter in SVO algorithms. CI, cardiac index; CO, cardiac output; FTc, systolic flow time corrected; HR, heart rate; PV, peak velocity; SVR, systemic vascular resistance.

Accuracy is an added advantage to Doppler techniques. At least 43 studies comparing the esophageal Doppler with the PAC suggest that the esophageal Doppler is as accurate as, or more accurate than, the PAC for cardiac output measurements.[25,26] The external Doppler's accuracy in measuring cardiac output has been validated against an aortic flow probe.[27]

Disadvantages
A limitation of the esophageal Doppler is that often patients must be sedated and usually intubated. When the user attempts to reacquire an adequate Doppler signal, any probe twisting or adjustment of probe depth is best tolerated with sedation. However, sedation is not required for the external Doppler. Although the sternal notch approach may be more likely to induce a cough in an intubated patient, signal acquisition is easy with the parasternal approach.

Supporting literature
Nine RCTs[9–17] using the esophageal Doppler mentioned earlier, as well as other patient outcome studies, have been the focus of technology reviews and systematic reviews of the literature published by the AHRQ,[28] NHS,[18] Centers for Medicare and

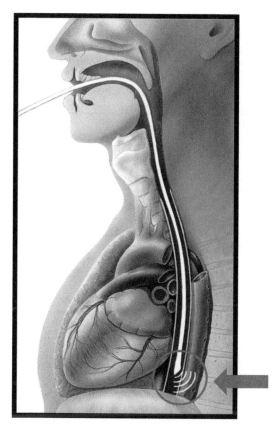

Fig. 5. Esophageal Doppler probe inserted to depth of approximately 30–40 cm (about T$_5$-T$_6$). Probe is twisted until the ultrasound beam at the end of the probe (illustrated by *red circle* and *arrow*) is directed at descending thoracic aorta, thus creating an aortic pulse wave. (*Reproduced* with kind permission from Deltex Medical, Chichester, UK.)

Medicaid Services,[29] and other third-party payers.[30] These articles consistently concluded that esophageal Doppler use was recommended for fluid optimization for perioperative patients and intubated patients in the ICU. At present, no cardiac output monitoring technique is supported by more evidence. However, more research is needed for the use of the esophageal Doppler in medical ICU populations such as patients with sepsis. Patient outcome studies regarding the use of the external (eg, noninvasive) Doppler are also ongoing. Although the external Doppler and the esophageal Doppler incorporate similar ways of measuring hemodynamic values, the external Doppler method requires more study in the critically ill patient population (3 of the 9 esophageal Doppler RCTs that suggested improved patient outcomes with SVO had conflicts of interest to disclose).[11,12,16]

Summary of Doppler techniques
Use of Doppler techniques provides the clinician with several advantages (**Table 2**). Minimally invasive applications, ease of use (esophageal Doppler), and accuracy are distinct strengths. However, no hemodynamic monitoring device is perfect for all

Table 2
Case study: a 56-year-old man is 30 minutes after coronary artery bypass grafting with bypass pump assist; a 200-mL increase in chest tube output is observed during the last hour; coagulation studies are pending; esophageal Doppler peak velocity reading is normal at 76 cm/s

Intervention/ Observation	Time	HR (bpm)	BP (mm Hg)	PAP (mm Hg)	CVP (mm Hg)	SV (mL)	FTc (ms)	CI (L/min/m²)	Svo₂ (%)[a]
Increase in chest tube output noted: 250 mL of 5% albumin IV bolus initiated	1200	88	113/72	26/13	8	49	282	2.2	57
Response to bolus noted. Another 250 mL of 5% albumin IV bolus started	1215	87	118/74	28/15	8	66	302	2.6	68
Response to bolus noted. Another 250 mL of 5% albumin IV bolus started	1230	88	123/78	29/17	8	74	337	2.9	73
Response to bolus noted. CT output decreased. Coagulation studies normal. Continue to monitor; no further fluid challenges indicated	1245	85	121/77	28/16	9	76	338	3.0	74

Volume challenges were stopped appropriately at 1245 because the SV and CI stopped responding by 10% or more after the third IV bolus of albumin. Note that the CVP remained essentially unchanged.

Abbreviations: BP, blood pressure; bpm, beats per minute; CI, cardiac index; CT, chest tube; CVP, central venous pressure; FTc, systolic flow time corrected (normal = 330–360 ms); HR, heart rate; PAP, pulmonary artery pressure.

[a] Normal Svo₂ is 60% to 80%.

patients in all situations, and any device used for monitoring has limitations. For example, the esophageal Doppler often requires the patient to be sedated.

Pulse Contour Method

The concept that cardiac output can be measured from an arterial line has existed for approximately 100 years. Otto Frank[31] (of the Frank-Starling curve) described the ability to measure cardiac output from the arterial line in 1899. Shortly thereafter, in 1904, Erlanger and Hooker[32] described that cardiac output was proportional to the arterial pulse pressure. Although the pulse contour monitors are new, the physiologic principles on which they are based are long-standing.

Description

Pulse contour techniques derive hemodynamic values in different ways via calculations of area under the curve for the systolic arterial pulse waveform. These calculations are based on the concept that pulse pressure and SV vary over the course of the respiratory cycle (pulsus paradoxus principle). During a normal inhalation, the diaphragm drops, intrathoracic pressure decreases, and the subsequent fluid volume gradient causes right ventricular venous return to increase. During exhalation, intrathoracic pressure increases as the diaphragm recoils and slightly compresses the mediastinal structures. This recoil facilitates an emptying of the pulmonary venous system and increases left ventricular filling.[33] This intrathoracic pressure gradient (and the influence on cardiac filling) is reversed when a patient is on positive pressure mechanical ventilation. However, these predictable patterns in blood flow and pulse pressure variation (PPV) during the respiratory cycle form the basis by which pulse contour techniques derive their values and may be used to predict fluid responsiveness in mechanically ventilated hypovolemic patients.

These blood flow patterns are also predictable enough to derive mathematical formulas from them. Each commercially available pulse contour device uses different proprietary software and mathematical algorithms to calculate similar hemodynamic values. The exact mathematical formulas are outside the scope of this article because of their complexity. However, they all calculate cardiac output and the dynamic parameters of PPV and/or SV variation (SVV).

In theory, calculations for PPV and SVV are simple. For example, pulse pressure (systolic blood pressure − diastolic blood pressure) is indirectly proportional to arterial compliance (AC) (PP = 1/AC), and pulse pressure is directly proportional to SV (PP $\propto$ SV). Pulse pressure also varies during the ventilator cycle (particularly during late inspiration of a ventilator-assisted breath), and PPV may help to predict recruitable cardiac output to fluid challenges. It is generally accepted that PPV of greater than or equal to 13% is predictive of identifying a fluid responder.[34] However, studies validating the impact of PPV and SVV on patient outcomes such as mortality and length of stay are still needed.

SVV also varies during the respiratory cycle and the degree of variability is expressed as a percentage:

$$[(SV_{maximum} - SV_{minimum} \times 100)/SV_{mean}]$$

An increasing amount of data suggests that volume-depleted patients may generate a higher degree of SVV.[35,36]

SVV greater than 13% may suggest that a fluid challenge will increase cardiac output; SVV less than 13% may suggest that a fluid challenge will not increase cardiac output.

Techniques

Three primary manufacturers exist for pulse contour continuous cardiac output monitors: lithium dilution cardiac output (LiDCO) (LiDCO Ltd, England), pulse contour cardiac output (PiCCO) (Pulsion Medical Systems, Germany), and FloTrac (Edwards Lifesciences, Irvine, CA). All calculate similar values by use of slightly different algorithms.

LiDCO uses transpulmonary indicator dilution to measure cardiac output by using lithium as the indicator. A trace dose of lithium is injected via a central or peripheral vein and the ion washout is detected by a sensor attached to an arterial line. LiDCO calculates SVV, PPV, cardiac output, and SV. The limitations of this technique are as follows: contraindication in patients already receiving lithium therapy, decreased accuracy in patients on muscle relaxant infusions, and decreased accuracy in patients with dysrhythmias.

PiCCO also calculates SVV, PPV, cardiac output, and SV. However, as opposed to LiDCO, PiCCO uses 15 to 20 mL of cold saline as its transpulmonary dilution indicator. Patients monitored with PiCCO also require central venous access as well as a central arterial (brachial or femoral) line to facilitate calculating an area under the curve to determine cardiac output. Both LiDCO and PiCCO require calibration by the clinician at regular intervals to maintain accurate values.

FloTrac may be the easiest pulse contour technique to use, because it requires only an arterial line, no lithium, and it autocalibrates. However, unlike LiDCO and PiCCO, FloTrac does not display PPV and generates an SVV value instead.

Advantages
Convenience may be an advantage for providers considering using pulse contour techniques for patients who already require arterial lines. Another perceived advantage is that the patient does not have to be intubated.

Disadvantages
Significant disadvantages may seem to outweigh the advantages of pulse contour techniques. These disadvantages include:

1. The need for invasive lines (arterial line; PiCCO requires central venous access as well).
2. Documented inaccuracies of hemodynamic values in the presence of dysrhythmias, atrial fibrillation, spontaneous mechanical ventilation,[37] low cardiac output states, low systemic vascular resistance states, very high or low cardiac output states, ventilator tidal volumes less than 8 mL/kg, low pulmonary compliance (ie, acute respiratory distress syndrome),[38] abrupt changes in hemodynamics,[39] and high or changing doses of vasopressors.[40,41]
3. Changes in vascular tone. As the vasculature changes, the physiologic algorithms in the software fail to adjust, thereby predisposing the system to inaccuracies.

Additional trends in evidence-based medicine increase the challenge of identifying a suitable candidate for pulse contour monitoring. For example, spontaneous mechanical ventilation is more frequent caused by trends toward minimizing sedation[42] and the recommendation for smaller tidal volumes to reduce the risk of ventilator-induced lung injury.

Supporting literature
A meta-analysis of 29 studies (n = 685) was performed to determine the ability of arterial waveform-derived variables to predict fluid responsiveness compared with static variables (eg, CVP, PAOP). The area under the receiver operating characteristic (ROC) curves were 0.94 for PPV and 0.84 for SVV (with 1 being the ideal predictive value) compared with an ROC of 0.55 for the CVP.[43] This study deserves recognition. However, RCTs focusing on patient outcomes are needed to further validate the role of pulse contour methods in hemodynamic optimization.

Evidence-based guidelines highly consider accumulation of RCTs when determining the strength of recommendations and assigning levels of evidence for given treatments. In contrast with the 9 RCTs suggesting patient benefit with esophageal Doppler techniques, the supporting evidence for pulse contour techniques is less robust. After an extensive literature search, the authors could find only 3 pulse contour RCTs (1 each for LiDCO,[44] PiCCO,[45] and the FloTrac method[46]) showing similar benefit (ie, length of stay) to that observed in the esophageal Doppler studies. All 3 studies disclosed conflicts of interest in the form of industry funding (grant to conduct study, consultant fees, speakers bureau, and so forth). However, 2 pulse contour

RCTs suggested no patient benefit (FloTrac[47] and PiCCO[48]). Therefore, more consistent research is needed to verify that care with the pulse contour method can produce the favorable patient outcome data that have been generated with esophageal Doppler studies.

Summary
Pulse contour techniques are increasing in popularity. However, the lack of consistent patient outcome data, invasiveness, and clinical factors that may contribute to inaccuracy should give clinicians pause. Further research will help to determine the clinical utility of pulse contour methods in the critically ill patient population.

Bioimpedance and Bioreactance

The concept of transmitting an electrical signal through tissue to obtain information for patient monitoring has existed for many years. Electrocardiogram monitoring is perhaps the best example. Bioimpedance and bioreactance operate under the same general principle; however, they conduct electrical signals through the entire thorax and obtain hemodynamic data. These techniques involve attaching electrodes on the neck, chest, and abdomen. By measuring the impedance thresholds between the electrodes during the cardiac cycle, values regarding blood flow and fluid volume status can be derived.

Description
Electrical current flows very efficiently through fluids and blood. However, air and tissue such as fat and bone are poorer conductors. Via electrodes placed on the neck and chest, bioimpedance and bioreactance measure the ability of the electricity to flow through the thorax and associated tissues as blood flows through the aorta and pulmonary vasculature throughout systole and diastole. The intrathoracic blood volume changes with each cardiac cycle can be used to indirectly determine SV, cardiac output, and other hemodynamic indices.

Techniques
The 2 primary techniques on the market are the Bio-Z (SonoSite, San Diego, CA) for bioimpedance and the non-invasive cardiac output monitor (NICOM) (Cheetah Medical, Vancouver, WA) for bioreactance. Bioreactance is a newer, second-generation technology that was designed to minimize the signal interference observed with the original bioimpedance signal quality (eg, signal/noise ratio). As a result, bioimpedance is sometimes referred to as amplitude modulation (AM) and bioreactance as frequency modulation (FM).

Advantages
The primary advantage of these techniques is the noninvasive application that enables clinicians to use them in a variety of inpatient and outpatient settings.

Disadvantages
Bioimpedance and bioreactance have struggled to establish themselves in critical care for several reasons. Signal acquisition is difficult in patients with large body habitus. The algorithms for calculating cardiac output are negatively affected by patient situations common in the critical care environment, such as motion artifacts, dysrhythmias, fluid overload, pleural effusions, and diaphoresis.

Supporting literature
More research is needed regarding the usefulness of bioimpedance and bioreactance in critical care. In 2012, Fagnoul and colleagues[49] published a bioreactance cardiac

output accuracy and comparison study with a semicontinuous thermodilution PAC (n = 11). Cardiac output measurements were obtained at study inclusion and after any relevant change in hemodynamic status, such as spontaneous changes in hemodynamics, during fluid bolus, or during titration of vasoactive agents. The study was terminated early because of poor correlation between PAC and bioreactance cardiac outputs (r = 0.145). At times, the bioreactance and PAC cardiac output values trended in opposite directions.

However, a recent article was more positive regarding bioreactance. In that study on the reliability of bioreactance with PLR in critical care, Marik and colleagues[50] compared bioreactance with carotid Doppler flow readings in a sample size (n = 34) that included sepsis/septic shock, patients on vasopressors, mechanically ventilated patients, and nonventilated patients. A strong correlation was found between the percentage change in SV index by PLR and the concomitant percentage change in carotid blood flow (r = 0.59, P = .0003). Sensitivity and specificity were 94% and 86%, respectively. Further research is needed to determine the clinical utility of bioreactance and the potential impact on patient outcomes.

Summary

Because of their noninvasive application, bioimpedance and bioreactance maintain popularity and remain intriguing alternatives to the PAC. Further study is needed to validate their accuracy and reliability in critical care. Most importantly, studies are still needed to establish this technology's effects on patient outcome.

Exhaled CO_2 Method and Capnometry

Exhaled CO_2 method

A newer application is the exhaled CO_2 method. This technique simply measures the amount of exhaled CO_2 and incorporates that into the Fick equation to calculate cardiac output. This method requires intubation and controlled mechanical ventilation and stable CO_2 elimination to be accurate. Heavy sedation or neuromuscular blockade are ideal to obtain accurate readings, which may prompt clinicians in the operating room to consider this technique, because deep sedation is generally discouraged in the intensive care setting unless medically necessary.[42] More research is needed regarding the exhaled CO_2 method.

Capnometry

Unlike the exhaled CO_2 method, waveform capnometry produces a measured end-tidal CO_2 (EtCO$_2$) value via infrared spectroscopy that can be used as a surrogate for cardiac output, rather than a derived, calculated cardiac output value.[51] A multitude of studies suggest that capnometry is helpful in assessing the adequacy of ventilation. However, the success of measuring ventilation in this way is predicated on the physiologic assertion that there is adequate right ventricular cardiac output to the lungs. As a result, changes in capnometry values in critical care may indicate concomitant changes in cardiac output when minute ventilation remains unchanged (**Fig. 6**).[51]

In a recent study (n = 65) of ventilated patients in the ICU, fluid-induced changes in EtCO$_2$ and cardiac index were well correlated (r = 0.45, P = .0001).[52] A PLR-induced increase in EtCO$_2$ greater than or equal to 5% predicted a fluid-induced increase in cardiac index greater than or equal to 15% with sensitivity of 71% and specificity of 100%. That finding suggests that changes in EtCO$_2$ induced by a PLR test can reliably predict fluid responsiveness. Research in this area is increasing. The area under the ROC curve for the PLR-induced changes in arterial pulse pressure was not significantly different from 0.5 (random chance probability).

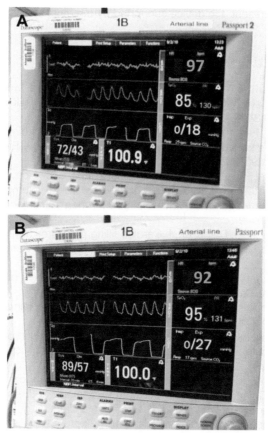

Fig. 6. (A) Pre–fluid challenge capnogram. A patient with septic shock is intubated in the field and is seen 15 minutes after arrival to the emergency department. A progressive decrease in $EtCO_2$ is observed to 18 mm Hg, followed by a decrease in blood pressure to 72/43 mm Hg. A 1-L 0.9% normal saline (NS) fluid challenge is initiated via pressure bag. (B) Post–fluid challenge capnogram. The 1-L 0.9% NS fluid challenge infused over 20 minutes and is now complete. Blood pressure has increased to 89/57 mm Hg; however, note the increase in $EtCO_2$ to 27 mm Hg. Minute ventilation remained unchanged at 8 L/min throughout the fluid challenge, which suggests that $EtCO_2$ was an indication of fluid responsiveness and may be used as a surrogate parameter for cardiac output.

SUMMARY

As discussed in this article, all current cardiac output monitoring devices have individual strengths and limitations, and no single device is best for all patients in all situations. However, all the devices discussed have indices for preload, afterload, and contractility in order to optimize SV and should trend similarly with respect to cardiac output, cardiac index, and SV. For example, in hypovolemia, cardiac output, cardiac index, and SV should all decrease similarly no matter what monitoring technique is used.

Regardless of the device chosen, an SVO algorithm approach should be considered, and volume challenges should be guided by assessments of fluid responsiveness. Although SVO requires further study in extubated and medical ICU populations, mortality benefit has been observed in high-risk surgical patients,[53,54] and we assert that SVO is supported by more evidence than CVP for fluid resuscitation. At present, the device supported by the most evidence is the esophageal Doppler.

REFERENCES

1. Marik P, Baram M, Vahid B. Does central venous pressure predict fluid responsiveness? A systematic review of the literature and the tale of seven mares. Chest 2008;134(1):172–8.
2. Benington S, Ferris P, Nirmalan M. Emerging trends in minimally invasive haemodynamic monitoring and optimization of fluid therapy. Eur J Anaesthesiol 2009;26(11):893–905.
3. Kumar A, Anel R, Bunnell E, et al. Pulmonary artery occlusion pressure and central venous pressure fail to predict ventricular filling volume, cardiac performance, or the response to volume infusion in normal subjects. Crit Care Med 2004;32(3):691–9.
4. Osman D, Ridel C, Ray P, et al. Cardiac filling pressures are not appropriate to predict hemodynamic response to volume challenge. Crit Care Med 2007;35(1): 64–8.
5. Marik P, Monnet X, Teboul JL. Hemodynamic parameters to guide fluid therapy. Ann Intensive Care 2011;1(1):1–9.
6. Turner M. Doppler-based hemodynamic monitoring. A minimally invasive alternative. AACN Clin Issues 2003;14(2):220–31.
7. Hamilton-Davies C, Mythen M, Salmon J, et al. Comparison of commonly used clinical indicators of hypovolaemia with gastrointestinal tonometry. Intensive Care Med 1997;23(3):276–81.
8. American College of Surgeons. Advanced trauma life support for doctors, ATLS. 8th edition. Chicago: American College of Surgeons; 2008.
9. Chytra I, Pradl R, Bosman R, et al. Esophageal Doppler-guided fluid management decreases blood lactate levels in multiple-trauma patients: a randomized controlled trial. Crit Care 2007;11(1):1–9.
10. Conway DH, Mayall R, Abdul-Latif MS, et al. Randomized controlled trial investigating the influence of intravenous fluid titration using esophageal Doppler monitoring during bowel surgery. Anesthesia 2002;57(9):845–9.
11. Gan TJ, Soppitt A, Maroof M, et al. Goal-directed intra-operative fluid administration reduces length of hospital stay after major surgery. Anesthesiology 2002; 97:820–6.
12. McKendry M, McGloin H, Saberi D, et al. Randomized controlled trial assessing the impact of a nurse delivered, flow monitored protocol for optimization of circulatory status after cardiac surgery. BMJ 2004;329(7460):258–61.
13. Mythen MG, Webb AR. Peri-operative plasma volume expansion reduces the incidence of gut mucosal hypoperfusion during cardiac surgery. Arch Surg 1995;130:423–9.
14. Sinclair S, James S, Singer M. Intraoperative intravascular volume optimization and length of hospital stay after repair of proximal femoral fracture: randomized controlled trial. BMJ 1997;315:909–12.
15. Venn R, Steele A, Richardson P, et al. Randomized controlled trial to investigate influence of the fluid challenge on duration of hospital stay and perioperative morbidity in patients with hip fractures. Br J Anaesth 2002;88:65–71.
16. Wakeling HG, McFall MR, Jenkins CS, et al. Intraoperative esophageal Doppler guided fluid management shortens postoperative hospital stay after major bowel surgery. Br J Anaesth 2005;95(5):634–42.

17. Noblett S, Snowden C, Shenton B, et al. Randomized clinical trial assessing the effect of Doppler-optimized fluid management on outcome after elective colorectal resection. Br J Surg 2006;93:1069–76.
18. Mowatt G, Houston G, Hernández R, et al. Systematic review of the clinical effectiveness and cost-effectiveness of oesophageal Doppler monitoring in critically ill and high-risk surgical patients. Health Technol Assess 2009;13(7):iii–iv, 1–134.
19. Cavallaro F, Sandroni C, Marano C, et al. Diagnostic accuracy of passive leg raising for prediction of fluid responsiveness in adults: systematic review and meta-analysis of clinical studies. Intensive Care Med 2010;36(9): 1475–83.
20. Thiel S, Kollef M, Isakow W. Non-invasive stroke volume measurement and passive leg raising predict volume responsiveness in medical ICU patients: an observational cohort study. Crit Care 2009;13(4):R111.
21. Monnet X, Rienzo M, Osman D, et al. Passive leg raising predicts fluid responsiveness in the critically ill. Crit Care Med 2006;34:1402–7.
22. Connors A, Speroff T, Dawson N, et al. The effectiveness of right heart catheterization in the initial care of critically ill patients. SUPPORT Investigators. JAMA 1996;276(11):889–97.
23. Balk E, Raman G, Chung M, et al. Evaluation of the evidence on benefits and harms of pulmonary artery catheter use in critical care settings. AHRQ Technology Assessment Report. 2008 [Internet] [cited September 21, 2013]. Available at: http://www.cms.gov/Medicare/Coverage/DeterminationProcess/downloads/id55TA.pdf. Accessed June 19, 2014.
24. Rajaram SS, Desai NK, Kalra A, et al. Pulmonary artery catheters for adult patients in intensive care [review]. Cochrane Database Syst Rev 2013;(2). CD003408 [Internet] [cited 2013 September 21]. Available at: http://onlinelibrary.wiley.com/doi/10.1002/14651858.CD003408.pub3/pdf/abstract.
25. Dark P, Singer M. The validity of trans-esophageal Doppler ultrasonography as a measure of cardiac output in critically ill adults. Intensive Care Med 2004;30: 2060–6.
26. Schober P, Loer S, Schwarte L. Perioperative hemodynamic monitoring with transesophageal Doppler technology. Anesth Analg 2009;109:340–53.
27. Phillips R, Hood S, Jacobson B, et al. Pulmonary artery catheter (PAC) accuracy and efficacy compared with flow probe and transcutaneous Doppler (USCOM): an ovine cardiac output validation. Crit Care Res Pract 2012;2012:621496. http://dx.doi.org/10.1155/2012/621496.
28. Agency for Healthcare Research and Quality. Esophageal Doppler ultrasound-based cardiac output monitoring for real-time therapeutic management of hospitalized patients – a review [Internet]. 2007. CMS.gov website [cited February 14, 2010]. Available at: http://www.cms.hhs.gov/determinationprocess/downloads/id45TA.pdf.
29. Center for Medicare and Medicaid Services. CMS manual system. Pub 100–03 Medicare national coverage determinations. 2007 [Internet]. CMS.hhs.gov website [cited February 14, 2010]. Available at: http://www.cms.hhs.gov/Transmittals/Downloads/R72NCD.pdf.
30. Aetna Health Insurance. Clinical policy bulletin: esophageal Doppler monitoring [Internet]. 2009. Aetna.com website [cited February 14, 2010]. Available at: http://www.aetna.com/cpb/medical/data/700_799/0793.html.
31. Frank O. Die grundform des arteriellen pulses. Erste abhandlung. Mathematische analyse. Zeitschrift für Biologie 1899;37:485–526.

32. Erlanger J, Hooker D. An experimental study of blood pressure and of pulse pressure in man. John Hopkins Hospital Records 1904;12:145–378.

33. Pinsky MR. Cardiovascular issues in respiratory care. Chest 2005;128(5 Suppl 2):592S–7S.

34. Greenfield N, Balk R. Evaluating the adequacy of fluid resuscitation in patients with septic shock: controversies and future directions. Hosp Pract 2012;40(2): 147–57.

35. Michard F. Changes in arterial pressure during mechanical ventilation. Anesthesiology 2005;103:419–28.

36. Michard F. Stroke volume variation: from applied physiology to improved outcomes. Crit Care Med 2011;39(2):402–3.

37. Perner A, Faber T. Stroke volume variation does not predict fluid responsiveness in patients with septic shock on pressure support ventilation. Acta Anaesthesiol Scand 2006;50(9):1068–73.

38. Monnet X, Bleibtreu A, Ferré A, et al. Passive leg-raising and end-expiratory occlusion tests perform better than pulse pressure variation in patients with low respiratory system compliance. Crit Care Med 2012;40(1):152–7.

39. Böettger S, Pavlovic D, Gründling M, et al. Comparison of arterial pressure cardiac output monitoring with transpulmonary thermodilution in septic patients. Med Sci Monit 2010;16(3):PR1–7.

40. Metzelder S, Coburn M, Fries M, et al. Performance of cardiac output measurement derived from arterial pressure waveform analysis in patients requiring high-dose vasopressor therapy. Br J Anaesth 2011;106(6):776–84.

41. Meng L, Tran N, Alexander B, et al. The impact of phenylephrine, ephedrine, and increased preload on third-generation Vigileo-FloTrac and esophageal Doppler cardiac output measurements. Anesth Analg 2011;113(4):751–7.

42. Barr J, Fraser G, Puntillo K, et al. Clinical practice guidelines for the management of pain, agitation, and delirium in adult patients in the intensive care unit. Crit Care Med 2013;41:263–306.

43. Marik P, Cavallazzi R, Vasu T, et al. Dynamic changes in arterial waveform derived variables and fluid responsiveness in mechanically ventilated patients: a systematic review of the literature. Crit Care Med 2009;37:2642–7.

44. Pearse R, Dawson D, Fawcett J. Early goal-directed therapy after major surgery reduces complications and duration of hospital stay. A randomized, controlled trial. Crit Care 2005;9(6):R687–93.

45. Goepfert M, Richter H, Zu Eulenburg C, et al. Individually optimized hemodynamic therapy reduces complications and length of stay in the intensive care unit. A prospective, randomized controlled trial. Anesthesiology 2013;119:824–36.

46. Mayer J, Boldt J, Mengistu A, et al. Goal-directed intraoperative therapy based on autocalibrated arterial pressure waveform analysis reduces hospital stay in high-risk surgical patients: a randomized, controlled trial. Crit Care 2010;14: R18. http://dx.doi.org/10.1186/cc8875.

47. Van der Linden PJ, Dierick A, Wilmin S, et al. A randomized controlled trial comparing an intraoperative goal-directed strategy with routine clinical practice in patients undergoing peripheral arterial surgery. Eur J Anaesthesiol 2010; 27(9):788–93.

48. Szakmany T, Toth I, Kovacs Z, et al. Effects of volumetric vs. pressure-guided fluid therapy on postoperative inflammatory response: a prospective, randomized clinical trial. Intensive Care Med 2005;31:656–63.

49. Fagnoul D, Vincent JL, De Backer D. Cardiac output measurements using the bioreactance technique in critically ill patients. Crit Care 2012;16(6):460.

50. Marik P, Levitov A, Young A, et al. The use of bioreactance and carotid Doppler to determine volume responsiveness and blood flow redistribution following passive leg raising in hemodynamically unstable patients. Chest 2013;143(2): 364–70.
51. Johnson A, Schweitzer D, Ahrens T. Time to throw away your stethoscope? Capnography: evidence-based patient monitoring technology. J Radiol Nurs 2011; 30:25–34.
52. Monnet X, Bataille A, Magalhaes E, et al. End-tidal carbon dioxide is better than arterial pressure for predicting volume responsiveness by the passive leg raising test. Intensive Care Med 2013;39(1):93–100.
53. Cecconi M, Corredor C, Arulkumaran N, et al. Clinical review: goal-directed therapy – what is the evidence in surgical patients? The effect on different risk groups. Crit Care 2013;17(2):209.
54. Poeze M, Greve J, Ramsay G. Meta-analysis of hemodynamic optimization: relationship to methodological quality. Critical Care 2005;9(6):R771–9.

The Experience of Family Members of ICU Patients Who Require Extensive Monitoring: A Qualitative Study

Claudia DiSabatino Smith, PhD, RN, NE-BC[a],*, Kristi Custard, BSN, RN[b]

KEYWORDS

- Cardiovascular intensive care unit • Monitoring equipment • Qualitative research
- Family research • High-tech monitoring • Instruction • Preoperative education

KEY POINTS

- Complex, high-tech monitoring equipment has stormed hospital intensive care units (ICUs).
- Although hospitals have kept pace with securing more sensitive invasive and noninvasive devices for health care professionals to monitor and deliver therapy to critically ill patients, the same cannot be said for helping families to cope with the conundrum of new devices.
- Accompanied by the emergence of extensive monitoring technology is a growing gap between health care providers, who use the technology to care for critically ill patients, and the patients' family members, who strain to understand and cope with its use on their loved one.
- A mixed methods study using family research with a phenomenological approach (n = 5 families) was conducted to explore family members' perceptions about the extensive monitoring technology used on their critically ill family member after cardiac surgery, as experienced when family members initially visited the patient in the cardiovascular ICU.
- Five relevant themes emerged: overwhelmed by all of the machines; feelings of uncertainty; methods of coping; meaning of the numbers on the machines; and need for education.

INTRODUCTION

Family members of critically ill patients experience high levels of situational anxiety and stress when loved ones are hospitalized in intensive care units (ICUs). Several

Funding Sources: Baylor St Luke's Nursing Research Council (C.D. Smith); Nil (K. Custard).
Conflict of Interest: None.
[a] Baylor St Luke's Medical Center, 6720 Bertner Avenue, MC 4-278, Box 77, Houston, TX 77030, USA; [b] Cardiovascular Recovery Room, Baylor St Luke's Medical Center, 6720 Bertner Avenue, MC 4-278, Box 192, Houston, TX 77030, USA
* Corresponding author.
E-mail address: Csmith1@StLukesHealth.org

Crit Care Nurs Clin N Am 26 (2014) 377–388
http://dx.doi.org/10.1016/j.ccell.2014.04.004
0899-5885/14/$ – see front matter © 2014 Elsevier Inc. All rights reserved.

factors are associated with this stress. Situational anxiety arises from worry about the patient's suffering and impending death, from concern about procedures, possible complications, and the equipment used in the care of the patient.[1] Over the last few years, complex, high-tech monitoring equipment has stormed hospital ICUs. Although hospitals have kept pace with securing more sensitive invasive and noninvasive devices for health care professionals to monitor and deliver therapy to critically ill patients, not the same can be said for helping families to cope with the conundrum of new devices. Accompanied by the emergence of this extensive monitoring technology is a growing gap between health care providers, who use the technology to care for critically ill patients, and the patients' family members, who strain to understand and cope with its use on their loved one.

As health care providers focus on monitoring screens, beeping alarms, and rows of neon numbers, family members watch with hopeful anticipation. The critical care experience personally affects family members; it may affect their own health and well-being, depending on the actions of the health care team and whether the family members' needs have been met. Understanding family members' perceptions of the high-tech monitoring equipment used on their loved one is one strategy to meet their needs. The purpose of this study was to explore family members' perceptions about the extensive monitoring technology used on their critically ill family member after cardiac surgery, as experienced when family members initially visited the patient in the cardiovascular ICU.

DEFINITION

For purposes of this study, high-tech, extensive monitoring is defined as continuous monitoring that goes beyond the standard ICU monitoring that consists of heart rate and rhythm, oxygen saturation, invasive and noninvasive blood pressure, and mechanical ventilator. High-tech, extensive monitoring includes the use of specialized equipment that not only monitors the patient but may also provide therapy to a subset of complex patients. In addition to the standard ICU monitoring, extensive monitoring includes hemodynamic monitoring, central venous pressure monitoring, or the use of one or more of the following: left ventricular assist devices (LVAD), hemodialysis (HD), continuous venovenous HD, continuous renal replacement therapy, and intra-aortic balloon pumps.

LITERATURE REVIEW
Family Member Communication

Family members of critically ill patients often receive patient information from health care professionals and share the information with other members of the family. They use the information to make treatment decisions for their loved ones based on their understanding.[2] Communication between health care providers and patients' families is important when determining treatment preferences and when conveying assessments and treatment plans.[3] Most communication between nurses and patients' families is in the biopsychosocial domain, when nurses talk with them about the patient's acute biomedical problems.[3] Little conversation occurs between nurses and patients' families in the domains of sharing power and responsibility when families are involved in decision making and the plan of care or when the patient is involved in the plan of care.[3] Family members experience added distress in situations when there is poor communication,[4,5] which may result from the inability to understand information, recall information, or receive information.[6]

Communication is a major component of patient-centered care and has been identified by patients' families as a critical aspect of high-quality ICU care.[3] Family members of critically ill patients need to receive updated information more than once to decrease anxiety.[4] Informative brochures that contain the contact information of health care representatives enable families to obtain information and provide them with the opportunity for more effective communication, which may reduce family members' distress and promote better comprehension.[6] Improving family communication is important, because time spent communicating with families adds to the already high costs of an ICU stay.[6] More than 50% of ICU patients' family members are at moderate to high risk for developing psychological distress long after the discharge or death of the patient.[7] Psychological distress includes depression, anxiety, and posttraumatic stress disorder (PTSD). Those who receive incomplete information are more likely to suffer from symptoms of PTSD.[8] Implementing proactive approaches to communication with family members decreases the occurrence of anxiety, depressive symptoms, and PSTD.[5]

Family Needs

Families of ICU patients have specific needs,[9] which are often left unmet.[10,11] The lack of attention to the needs of family members affects clinical outcomes and resource utilization in the ICU setting.[7]

Many family members experience symptoms of acute stress disorder when a loved one is admitted to the ICU.[8] Situational anxiety in family members may persist for as long as 72 hours after admission, although 73% of family members (n = 544) reported anxiety for as long as 9 days after a family member's admission to ICU.[1]

Because they are surrogate decision makers, the decisions that family members make affect not only the patient but also the family members.[7] The uncertainty that accompanies critical illness, coupled with communication barriers and fear, add to the distress levels of family members. In one study,[8] 81% of family members who participated in making end-of-life decisions experienced PTSD.

Family members of ICU patients reported that their greatest need was for information about the patient's status and about the equipment being used.[8] Strategies to help meet the needs of family members include reflective inquiry, which is looking back and clarifying for the family what happened, as well as family inclusion in the patient's plan of care.[12,13] The most important factor affecting the overall satisfaction of family members of ICU patients is the thoroughness of the information they receive.[4,14] Studies suggest that nurses should ask family members about their needs, rather than basing interventions on presumptions about those needs.[9,15,16] By understanding family members' perceptions of the high-tech monitoring equipment in use on the critically ill patient, nurses and doctors can tailor written materials to meet the knowledge deficit of family members.

Family members need to receive information about the equipment in use and the reason for the equipment. Strategies to improve the communication between health care providers and patients' family members should include not only implementing early, frequent family conferences but also assigning a liaison for the family. As family members describe their perceptions about the monitoring equipment being used on their critically ill loved one, the level of situational anxiety should be considered. The family members' level of anxiety may affect their perceptions as they relate to verbal and written instructions and education materials provided by health care providers. Therefore, additional insight may be gained by evaluating family members' level of stress at the time of the study interview. To supplement verbal instruction and to provide tailored, written materials that educate family members regarding extensive high-tech monitoring equipment, we need to understand the family's perceptions related to the equipment. Literature supports the need to increase and improve communication between health care professionals and the patients' families.

However, little is written about the family members' perceptions of the extensive, high-tech monitoring equipment used on their loved one.

THEORETIC FRAMEWORK

Critical illness causes a disruption in life.[17] In her grand theory, Sister Calista Roy refers to critical illness as a disruptive event that requires a period of adjustment, which is called the compensatory process. Adaptation to the event occurs after the period of adjustment. The events of the adjustment period determine if the outcome of adaptation is positive, negative, complete, or incomplete. The process of adaptation is an iterative process, and as the patient's condition changes, the patient's family must continue to adapt to the changes.

One strategy to assist patients' families to adapt to the changing patient condition is to provide timely, accurate, and consistent information to family members in an attempt to optimize the families' experience.[18] Surrogate decision makers need to be provided with early, effective communication[2] to inform decision making. Nurses can help family members who are in the compensatory process to move toward positive adaptation by using a thorough, structured approach to providing family information and support.[16]

The family's need for accurate information about the patient and the equipment is well documented in the literature, although little has been written on the family members' perceptions regarding the high-tech monitoring used on their critically ill loved one. A clearer understanding of family members' perceptions regarding the use of the monitoring equipment enables health care professionals to develop effective, tailored instructional materials, which may facilitate the adaptation of family members and reduce their situational anxiety and stress.

STUDY DESIGN

The researchers used a mixed methods study, using both quantitative and qualitative research, to answer the research questions. Individual family members provided informed consent in accordance with approval by the hospital Institutional Review Board. The Spielberger State Trait Anxiety Inventory (STAI)[19] measured the level of anxiety in participating family members. The qualitative arm of the study used a hermeneutic interpretive phenomenological approach to explore the family members' experience with high-tech monitoring equipment that was used with their loved one.

Research questions were:

1. What was the experience of family members who visited a critically ill loved one who was extensively monitored using high-tech monitoring equipment in the cardiovascular ICU after cardiac surgery?
2. What was the anxiety level of family members/the family at the time that they described their experience with their extensively monitored critically ill patient?
3. What information did family members of critically ill patients who were extensively monitored using high-tech monitoring equipment perceive that they received regarding the equipment used to monitor the patient?
4. What was the family members' perception regarding verbal and written information given to them that taught them about the equipment and care provided in the cardiovascular recovery room.

QUALITATIVE METHODOLOGY

Purposive sampling was used to recruit a sample of study participants, family members, who were identified by the cardiovascular ICU assistant nurse manager during visitation with patients after cardiac surgery. An effort was made to recruit a representative sample of study participants, although the researchers were not able to realize this goal. The limitation is further discussed later.

A semistructured interview guide was used, beginning with broad, grand-tier research questions and moving to smaller, lower-tier questions.[20] Sample questions include: (1) describe for me what you saw when you entered the room to see the patient after surgery; (2) tell me what you were thinking when you saw the patient connected to the machines and monitors; and (3) what instruction did the nurses/doctors give you about the monitors and machines?

Hermeneutic Phenomenology

Hermeneutics focuses on using people's lived experiences as a tool to understand the context in which those experiences occur. Phenomenology is the study of human experience from the perspective of those experiencing a particular phenomenon. The goal of hermeneutic phenomenological research is to enter another person's world to discover the practical wisdom, understanding, and possibilities associated with their experience.[21] Phenomenologists approach each interview with openness, and rely primarily on in-depth interpretation.[22]

Family Research

"A family is a self-defined social unit whose members may be biologically or legally related and live together and who have a shared reality and ongoing formation of meaning...."[23] Collective family interviews are particularly appropriate when the family is facing an issue that may be manageable, randomly or externally imposed, and a challenge for the family as a whole.[23] In this study, individual families were interviewed in a group, with no more than 4 family members per family interview.

Family data are developed in interaction[24] and are not intended to capture the more private thoughts and opinions of members. The researcher anticipates that responses of family members are modified by the presence of others, because they act as a family member, not an individual. Individual insights are not superior to family data, just different, in contrast to the concern that family members can often stimulate interaction and enrich insights and disclosure. A good way to encourage family members is by saying, "I am interested in what every family member thinks about what I am about to ask. I'm interested in how your whole family is responding."

Family members interact not only with the researcher, but more importantly with each other. Differing views are aired, discussed, and, at times, argued. "A truly family description of being a family emerges, not as a homogenized whole but a complex interplay of the individual and collective."[25] The goal of qualitative family research is to create a description of the family phenomenon in question that is grounded in themes common to the experiences of families generally and that reflects the experiences of individual families, that is, across and within case description.[26] The use of the family research interview approach provides family members with an opportunity to talk about their perception of the extensive monitoring technology, which may facilitate their compensatory adaptation to the patient's changing condition.

QUANTITATIVE METHODOLOGY
Instruments

Two instruments provided quantitative data. A researcher-generated demographic data collection form was used to secure participants' age, gender, ethnicity, and relationship to the patient from every individual within the study families. The researchers did not collect information from the patients' medical record. The STAI was completed by each study participant at the inception of the group interviews. The STAI has been widely used to measure anxiety in adults.

Scores on the STAI anxiety scale increase in response to physical danger and psychological stress and decrease as a result of relaxation training.[27] In this self-report measure, patients are asked to complete a 40-item tool using a Likert scale. The questions are focused on their feelings of apprehension, tension, nervousness, and worry. Total scores obtained from the STAI range from 20 to 80. There are 2 separate self-report scales within the STAI that measure state (S) and trait (T). Spielberger described the "S-Anxiety scale as consisting of twenty statements that evaluate how respondents feel *right now*, at this moment and the T-Anxiety scale of twenty statements that assess how people *generally* feel."[19(p32)] Furthermore, when this instrument is administered immediately during a stressful situation, it has an α reliability of .92 to .94.[19] The correlations between state and trait anxiety scales for males and females in different population groups varied from 0.59 to 0.75.[19]

DATA ANALYSIS
Qualitative Data

The researchers analyzed the qualitative data before any quantitative analysis was undertaken to avoid researcher bias. Diekelmann (1989) in Polit and Beck (2012)[28] descriptive phenomenological method was used to analyze the interview data. Diekelmann's method includes elements of both descriptive and interpretive phenomenology. This method consists of a 7-phase process, which includes:

1. Read all the participants' descriptions of the phenomenon for an overall understanding.
2. Write interpretive summaries of each interview.
3. The research team analyzes select transcribed interviews or text.
4. Any disagreements on interpretation are resolved by going back to the text.
5. Common meanings are identified through comparison and contrast of the text.
6. Relationships among the themes emerge.
7. A draft of the themes with exemplars from the text is presented to the research team. Comments are incorporated into the final draft.[28]

As an additional step to ensure trustworthiness of the data, the principal investigator secured the services of a professional colleague who was familiar with qualitative research to review the interview transcripts and interpretive findings for accuracy and consistency.

Quantitative Data

After the completion of data analysis of the qualitative arm of the study, quantitative analysis was conducted to assess the anxiety level of each individual participant, as well as to determine a composite anxiety score for each family unit. Frequency tables were calculated for the demographic data and STAI scores. Resultant family anxiety composite scores were compared with qualitative findings to explore any relationships that may exist.

FINDINGS
Qualitative

Six general themes emerged from the analysis of 5 family interviews. One of the themes did not inform the research questions; it was, "the nurses are wonderful." Early in the group interviews, each of the participating families affirmed that the "nurses did a wonderful job" and "taught them all that they needed to know." However, as the interview progressed, families consistently admitted, "there were things that it would have been helpful to know." Therefore, relevant emerging themes were: overwhelmed by all of the machines; feelings of uncertainty; methods of coping; meaning of the numbers on the machines; and need for education. Excerpts from the transcriptions show justification for the theme selections.

Overwhelmed by all of the machines
- When we came into the room we saw, "all the monitors, you see the nurse's computer and then all of the monitors and all the wires, the tubing, the nurse...."
- "... a lot of bags of liquids, a lot of tubes... and really the size of the machines, like the bulk of it looked like he had 2 huge computer stations on both side[s] of him, tied into him. That's what we noticed."
- "Even though everybody told me what to expect and stuff, it was still worse than I thought it would be. Even in my worst imagination, it still was worse."
- "The tree with all of the pumps on it... 4 pumps per row, 3 rows, 12 different pumps.... That tree was a little bit more than what I've seen before. I normally see 2 or 3 machines after surgery, but this time she had a lot more; like the tree of pumps."

Feelings of uncertainty
- "I was wondering if the machines were doing all of the work for him, if he was doing any of the work for himself or if he was going to need that type of equipment for the rest of his life. I wondered if that was something that he would recover from. It didn't seem...it just looked like...how could he possibly recover from all of this?"
- "My worry was how long was he gonna be sedated. I know they were sedating on purpose, but was he gonna come out of the sedation?"

Methods of coping
- "I tend to focus on the blood pressure, the things that I'm familiar with. I don't really look around a lot. He was probably there a week before I noticed there was a sink in the room [where] I could wash my hands."
- "I just like asking each [staff member] person if they would tell me this again... I just like to look and point and say, what's that, and what's that?"
- "I looked at [patient name] lying there, and I'm thinking, I'm so happy and he's happy and I know he's in a lot of pain, but I just think how blessed we are that he got all of this and [they're] taking care of him. They didn't have all of this, years ago." "The other people were so generous to us. The other family so willingly gave everything that child had..."

Meaning of the numbers on the machines
- We saw "graphs, a lot of numbers, a lot of information that would seem to mean something, but you don't really understand what."
- "How do you know what the norm is? Do you know that that's a good number that you are looking at?"
- "...I didn't know what any of those numbers and things meant on that monitor that heart beating and blood pressure and I don't remember what any of the rest of them were...."
- "Each patient would have different parameters, but even if we just knew what each color and line meant and what it was measuring, I think that would have been very helpful." "...parameters of what you would expect for the heart beat, what good blood pressure numbers are, and maybe your oxygen saturation."

Need for education

- "I think the more education the earlier you have for the technology the better. That was the first thing I did… I've never heard of an LVAD before this and I went straight home and just spent hours just researching it and reading about other patients' experiences and the process of LVAD recovery. To maybe have that as reading material in the waiting room, or maybe have an iPad app that gives you… meet the hospital equipment. Meet the ventilation machine…and it gives you a breakdown of the ventilation machine and what the charts and graphs mean that you're looking at."
- "An app would be nice; an interactive one."
- In the doctor's office they "had pictures and showed what his [heart] looked like and what they were gonna do and what they were gonna repair, so that was very helpful. But they didn't have anything on the equipment." "They could just have… here's a picture of the monitors, and this is your heart rate; this is your blood pressure; this is this, I think that would have been very helpful."
- More education "gives you something to feel empowered, to feel like you have a little more control of the situation. But besides that, it would be helpful for family members who want to understand more about what is going on."
- It would have been helpful if they would "tell you what each little thing means….like what is patient saturation, what is the pulse, what is the breathing rate, the blood pressure. Not everybody knows that."
- "We were given a brochure on the LVAD device…and I went out and did a lot of research on my own to understand more about it. …the information that I got was formidable. I do believe that it's your personal responsibility to become educated in something that truly is a life-changing event…. I'll never be an expert, but I'll be knowledgeable and with knowledge comes power."

Quantitative

The study sample consisted of 71% female and 86.7% white family members. Of these individuals, 57% were spouses of the critically ill patient, whereas 14% were grandmother, 14% son, and 14% daughter of the patient. Ages ranged from 29 to 77 years, with an average age of 57.4 years. Seventy-one percent of the patients had 4 monitors/machines in addition to the standard monitoring devices, whereas 29% had 3 additional monitors/machines.

STAI scores suggested that both family members in 1 of 5 families fell in the high anxiety domain, whereas the remaining 4 families scored in the low to medium level. The small sample size limits any kind of generalization in terms of quantitative findings.

DISCUSSION

Study findings concur with those of Tracy and colleagues,[1] who suggested that situational anxiety arises from worry about the patient's suffering and from concern about the equipment used in the care of the patient. Several families talked about their conflicted feelings related to wanting their loved one to be relieved of pain, yet having concerns about their level of sedation and wondering " how long was he gonna be sedated… but was he gonna come out of the sedation?" Such worries may have been avoided had preoperative education about the use of sedation during mechanical ventilation, and the need for adequate pain relief, been provided. Family members validated findings of Alvarez and Kirby,[4] who said that family members need to receive updated information more than once to decrease anxiety. One spouse confided, "I just like asking each [staff member] person if they would tell me this again." She went on to say that she knew that she had asked previously, but she just could not remember the answers to her questions. Family members in this study admitted asking nurses repeatedly about the use of certain equipment and normal parameters of various vital statistics.

Literature supports the use of informative brochures to educate families about equipment in use and treatment regimens commonly used in critically ill patients.[6] Families in this study consistently reported that they received no informational brochures, aside from those who received information about the LVAD. A few family members reported that they preferred to obtain their information by talking to hospital staff members; some wanted written material that they could refer to later, whereas others suggested the development of interactive computer applications. Regardless of the vehicle in which the instruction is provided, all of the participants expressed the need for more education. Each of the themes that emerged from the study findings is a product of an overarching need for education. Families may not have been so overwhelmed by all of the machines if they had been introduced to them before encountering them attached to their loved one. They may not have had such feelings of uncertainty, or had difficulty coping if they had received instructional materials that showed the monitoring equipment in use in an ICU setting. Fundamental information related to a range of normal parameters for routine vital signs could go a long way to reducing anxiety related to the meaning of the numbers shown on the monitors.

Further, the literature[8] suggests that family members experience symptoms of acute stress disorder when a loved one is admitted to the ICU, although STAI scores in this study indicated high anxiety in only 20% of participating family members. The investigators suggested the possibility that some of the families who declined to participate in the study may have had higher levels of anxiety than those who agreed to participate.

Only 5 of the 6 emerging themes inform the research questions. The sixth theme, "the nurses are wonderful," may have been a heartfelt affirmation of the family members in regard to the nursing care experienced by the patient and family during the critical postoperative period. However, it is not relevant to the questions under study. Family members were quick to praise the nursing staff. One spouse said, "The nurses are wonderful! They always answer my questions." Another commented that, "I felt better once I realized that he would never be left alone; I mean a nurse would always be with him, even through the night."

One cannot overlook the possibility for bias, because all of the patients were in the cardiovascular ICU at the time of the interviews.

Research question 1 asks about the experience of families who visit patients with extensive monitoring equipment in the cardiovascular ICU. All but one of the families concurred with this family member's feeling about the experience. "Even though everybody told me what to expect and stuff, it was still worse than I thought it would be. Even in my worst imagination, it still was worse." The patient of the family who did not ascribe to this perception was a young man who had received a heart transplant. The patient's main caregiver said, "I looked at [patient name] lying there, and I'm thinking, I'm so happy and he's happy and I know he's in a lot of pain, but I just think how blessed we are that he got all of this and [they're] taking care of him." "... And he was thinking the same thing. We were so grateful, so very grateful."

Research question 2 explores the anxiety level of the family members at the time of the interview. As indicated earlier, only 20% of the families showed a high level of stress as measured by the STAI. However, at least 10 families who were approached to enroll in the study declined to do so. Several of them admitted to the coinvestigator that they were too stressed to participate "right now, maybe next week." Each was given the business card of the primary investigator, but none contacted the study team.

The third research question explores the perception of families regarding information that they received about the monitoring equipment. One family commented that in the doctor's office they "had pictures and showed what his [heart] looked like and what they were gonna do and what they were gonna repair, so that was very helpful. But they didn't have anything on the equipment." Another family member admitted that "We were given a brochure on the LVAD device" that his spouse received. All families concurred that none of them had received information about any of the cadre of extensive monitoring equipment. Most of the families agreed with the family member who said, "They could just have... here's a picture of the monitors, and this is your heart rate; this is your blood pressure; this is this, I think that would have been very helpful."

Research question 4 deals more directly with information provided in either verbal or written format about not only the monitoring equipment but also the patient care that is provided in a high-acuity cardiovascular surgery critical care unit. Family members consistently denied receiving any instructional materials, aside from the vendor-generated LVAD brochure. Despite one family member who had commented early in the interview that "the nurses told me all that I needed to know," they later admitted that "there were things that would have been nice to know."

Another had a similar comment, "It would have been helpful if they would tell you what each little thing means....like what is patient saturation, what is the pulse, what is the breathing rate, the blood pressure. Not everybody knows that." More than one family member suggested that if there were printed booklets about what to expect about ICU care and all of the equipment, they could have repeatedly referred to them throughout their loved one's ICU stay. Education not only answers questions but also "gives you something to feel empowered, to feel like you have a little more control of the situation. But besides that, it would be helpful for family members who want to understand more about what is going on."

This study concurs with Auerbach and colleagues,[8] who found that families need information about the patient's condition and the equipment that is being used in the patient's care. Family members' satisfaction with the patient care administered in the ICU can be increased by simply providing tailored instructional materials about the equipment and general care provided in the cardiovascular ICU, as suggested in previous studies.[4,14]

LIMITATIONS

The small number of participants and the lack of cultural diversity among the sample limit generalizability of the study findings. Despite efforts to recruit participants who were not white, only 1 Hispanic family participated in the study. Another limitation of the study may be the inclusion of 1 family in which the grandparents raised the patient who received a heart transplant, whereas the family members of the remaining 4 patients were spouses and children of patients who underwent nontransplant cardiovascular surgery. The grandparent-grandson relationship or receipt of a heart transplant versus nontransplant cardiovascular surgery may explain differences noted in the family member's responses that do not necessarily concur with that of other families. One such difference was the family's response when asked what they saw when they entered the room. My eyes "went right to that little face.... We realize the importance of this machinery that's keeping him comfortable and keeping his body going and everything. We were not shocked... he's not swollen like I thought he would be." The family also commented, "All I can say is I'm excited and I'm thankful and I'm grateful...."

All of the families were grateful for the vigilance of the nursing staff in caring for their loved one, but all agreed that they received little or no education about the high-tech monitoring equipment. Although anxiety levels in 80% of family members were in the bottom 50th percentile, 20% were higher than the 70th percentile. Family members would like to receive education about the equipment in use on their critically ill loved one, as well as about normal parameters of vital statistics, and 38% of family members would prefer interactive electronic education.

REFERENCES

1. Tracy J, Fowler S, Magarelli K. Hope and anxiety of individual family members of critically ill adults. Appl Nurs Res 1999;12:121–7.
2. Azoulay E, Sprung CL. Family-physician interactions in the intensive care unit. Crit Care Med 2004;32(11):2323–8.
3. Slatore CG, Hansen L, Ganzini L, et al. Communication by nurses in the intensive care unit: qualitative analysis of domains of patient-centered care. Am J Crit Care 2012;21(6):410–8.
4. Alverez GF, Kirby AS. The perspective of families of the critically ill patient: their needs. Curr Opin Crit Care 2006;12(6):614–8.
5. Jacobowski NL, Girard TD, Mulder JA, et al. Communication in critical care: family rounds in the intensive care unit. Am J Crit Care 2010;19(5):421–30.
6. Azoulay E, Chevert S, Leleu G, et al. Half the families of intensive care unit patients experience inadequate communication with physicians. Crit Care Med 2000;28(8):3044–9.
7. Hickman RL, Douglas SL. Impact of chronic critical illness on the psychological outcomes of family members. AACN Adv Crit Care 2010;21(1):80–91.
8. Auerbach SM, Kiesler DJ, Wartella J, et al. Optimism satisfaction with needs met, interpersonal perceptions of the healthcare team and emotional distress in patients' family members during critical care hospitalization. Am J Crit Care 2005;14:202–10.
9. Kleinpell RM, Powers MJ. Needs of family members of intensive care patients. Appl Nurs Res 1992;5(1):2–8.
10. Titler MG, Cohen MZ, Craft MJ. Impact of adult critical care hospitalization: perceptions of patients, spouses, children, and nurses. Heart Lung 1991;20(2):174–82.
11. Cuthbertson SJ, Margetts MA, Streat SJ. Bereavement follow-up after critical illness. Crit Care Med 2000;28(4):1196–201.
12. Melnyk BM, Alpert-Gillis L, Feinstein NF, et al. Creating opportunities for parent empowerment: program effects on the mental health/coping outcomes of critically ill young children and their mothers. Pediatrics 2004;113(6):597–607.
13. Weick KE. Making sense of the organization. Malden (MA): Blackwell; 2001.
14. Medina J. Natural synergy in creating a patient-focused care environment: the critical care family assistance program and critical care nursing. Chest 2005;128(Suppl 3):99–102.
15. Mi-kuen T, French P, Kai-kwong L. The needs of the family of critically ill neurosurgical patients: a comparison of nurses' and family members' perceptions. J Neurosci Nurs 1999;31(6):348–56.
16. Davidson JE. Family-centered care: meeting the needs of patients' families and helping families adapt to critical illness. Crit Care Nurse 2009;29(3):28–34.
17. Roy C, Andrews HA. The Roy adaptation model. Stamford (CT): Appleton & Lange; 1999.

18. Davidson JE, Powers K, Hedayat KM, et al. Clinical practice guidelines for support of the family in the patient-centered ICU: American College of Critical Care Task Force 2004-2005. Crit Care Med 2007;35(2):605–22.

19. Spielberger CD. State-Trait Anxiety Inventory (STAI) for adults manual and sample: manual, instrument and scoring guide. 1983. Available at: http://www.mindgarden.com/. Permission granted by MindGarden on August 3, 2012.

20. Marshall C, Rossman GB. Designing qualitative research. 4th edition. Thousand Oaks (CA): Sage; 2006.

21. Polit DF, Beck CT. Nursing research: generating and assessing evidence for nursing practice. 9th edition. Philadelphia: Wolters Kluwer/Lippincott Williams & Wilkins; 2012.

22. Lindseth A, Norberg A. A phenomenological hermeneutical method for researching lived experience. Scand J Caring Sci 2004;18(2):145–53.

23. Donalek JG. The family research interview. Nurse Researcher 2009;16(3):21–8.

24. Daly KJ. Family theory versus the theories families live by. J Marriage Fam 2003; 65(4):771–84.

25. Dahl CM, Boss P. The use of phenomenology for family therapy research: the search for meaning. In: Sprenkle DH, Piercy FP, editors. Research methods in family therapy. 2nd edition. New York: Guilford Press; 2005. p. 63–84.

26. Ayers L, Kavanaugh K, Knafl KA. Within-case and across-case approaches to qualitative data analysis. Qual Health Res 2003;13(6):871–83.

27. MindGarden. State-Trait Anxiety Inventory for adults. 2012. Purchased at: http://www.mindgarden.com/products/staisad.htm#about.

28. Diekelmann NL, Allen D, Tanner C. The NLN criteria for appraisal of baccalaureate programs: A critical hermeneutic analysis. In: Polit DF, Beck CT, editors. Nursing research: Generating and assessing evidence for nursing practice; 1989. p. 565–9.

Brain Perfusion and Oxygenation

Laura L. Lipp, MS, APRN, ACNP-BC, CNRN

KEYWORDS

- Brain perfusion and oxygenation • Oxygen consumption
- Cerebral metabolic rate of oxygen • Cerebral blood flow • Neuromonitoring

KEY POINTS

- Maintenance of brain perfusion and oxygenation is of paramount importance to patient outcome with various types of brain injuries (traumatic, ischemic, and hemorrhagic).
- Historically, monitoring of intracranial pressure (ICP) and cerebral perfusion pressure (CPP) has been the mainstay of neuromonitoring techniques used at the critical care bedside to monitor brain perfusion and oxygenation.
- Within recent years, other neuromonitoring techniques have been studied and developed to provide information concerning brain perfusion and oxygenation.

PHYSIOLOGY OF BRAIN PERFUSION AND OXYGENATION
Cerebral Metabolism

Cerebral metabolism is supported by the constant supply of oxygen and glucose.[1,2] Oxygen consumption by the brain accounts for approximately 20% of the total body oxygen consumption.[3] The cerebral metabolic rate of oxygen ($CMRO_2$) averages 3 to 3.8 mL/100 g/min. Neuronal electrical activity is supported through the generation of ATP, which requires approximately 60% of the total brain oxygen consumption.[1] Most of the ATP produced in the body is the result of oxidative phosphorylation occurring in the mitochondria of the cell, which is otherwise known as aerobic metabolism.[4] In cerebral metabolism, aerobic metabolism depends on the continuous presence of oxygen and glucose.[1,4]

Glucose is the primary source of energy in the brain.[1] This energy promotes maintenance of the gradient of ions across the cerebral cell membrane and transmission of electrical impulses.[3] The brain consumes glucose at the rate of 5 mg/100 g/min, mostly through aerobic metabolism. A continuous supply of glucose is necessary to maintain cerebral function.[1] Hypoglycemia can cause seizures and loss of consciousness.[5] Hyperglycemia can accelerate cerebral acidosis, which promotes cell damage

Conflict of Interest: Nil.
Nurse Practitioner Service, Houston Methodist Hospital, 6565 Fannin Street, Houston, TX 77030, USA
E-mail address: llipp@houstonmethodist.org

and can exacerbate brain injury.[1] Without the continuous presence of oxygen, aerobic metabolism changes to anaerobic metabolism, using the glucose present to produce ATP through the breakdown of glucose to pyruvate to lactate, which results in metabolic acidosis.[2,4]

If brain tissue perfusion is interrupted, with resulting hypoxia, ATP stores are reduced. Under most circumstances, if (cerebral blood flow CBF) is not reestablished within 3 to 8 min, irreversible cellular injury to cerebral tissue occurs.[1]

Decreased CBF results in hypoxia and ischemic injury to the cell. Potassium exits the cell and calcium enters the cell, causing cellular acidosis and necrosis of the cell. Glutamate, a neurotransmitter, is released by ischemic cells. Glutamate promotes the movement of sodium and calcium into the cell, thereby causing cellular edema. Inflammatory mediators (such as prostaglandins and leukotrienes) accumulate as a result of the ischemia and necrosis and cause cellular edema. Biochemical events, such as free radical production, caused by ischemia damage the cell membrane through peroxidation. These processes lead to cellular edema and cell death.[2]

CBF

As previously stated, the brain requires a constant perfusion to ensure the delivery of oxygen necessary for cellular metabolism.[1,6] Oxygen delivery to the brain is accomplished through normal CBF. On an average, the normal CBF is 54 mL/100 g/min in an average brain weighing 1400 g. In other words, normal CBF averages 756 mL/min.[3]

In traumatic brain injury, irreversible tissue damage occurs when the CBF threshold decreases to 15 mL/100 g/min. In ischemic stroke, irreversible tissue damage occurs when the CBF threshold decreases to 5 to 8.5 mL/100 g/min.[7] In general, cerebral impairment is associated with a CBF between 20 and 25 mL/100 g/min.[1]

Determinants of CBF

ICP is maintained through a mechanism known as the Monro-Kellie doctrine. The components of ICP are the brain, blood, and cerebrospinal fluid. If a component increases owing to injury, insult, or disease, then another component must decrease to maintain a stable ICP.[8] The normal ICP, in general, ranges between 5 and 10 mm Hg.[9] The general goal is to maintain the ICP less than 20 mm Hg.[6]

Autoregulation in the brain is a process whereby the CBF is maintained through vasodilation and vasoconstriction of cerebral arterioles to promote a constant CPP. Vasodilation occurs if the systemic blood pressure decreases to allow an increase in CBF. Vasoconstriction occurs if the systemic blood pressure increases, thereby decreasing CBF to prevent hyperperfusion.[3,6] Several factors influence autoregulation. Hypoxia, hyperthermia, acidosis, and hypoventilation cause vasodilation (increase in CBF). Hypothermia, alkalosis, and hyperventilation cause vasoconstriction (decrease in CBF).[9] Cerebral autoregulation can be impaired by insults such as trauma, hypoxemia, and hypercapnia.[7] When brain tissue is damaged by such insults, autoregulation is impaired and cerebral ischemia can result.[9]

Cerebral autoregulation directly affects CBF, thereby preserving CPP over a wide range of mean arterial blood pressure (60–160 mm Hg).[1,3,6] CPP is the difference between the mean arterial pressure (MAP) and the cerebral venous pressure, which is approximated by the ICP.[1,9] More clearly stated, CPP = MAP − ICP.[10] Guidelines for the management of severe traumatic brain injury promote the maintenance of CPP between 50 and 70 mm Hg. Cerebral ischemia may be a greater threat at levels less than 50 mm Hg. The development of adult respiratory distress syndrome is a greater risk at levels greater than 70 mm Hg.[11]

CBF, arterial oxygen content, and $CMRO_2$ are the determinative factors for cerebral oxygenation. CPP is the most frequently used surrogate for CBF. However, it is recommended to monitor cerebral oxygenation and metabolism to achieve individualized therapy while maintaining the CPP between 50 and 70 mm Hg.[7]

Respiratory gas tensions affect CBF. For example, the $Paco_2$ has a profound effect. For $Paco_2$ tensions between 20 and 80 mm Hg, a direct proportionate effect can be seen. As $Paco_2$ increases, cerebral vasodilation occurs, with an increase in CBF. As $Paco_2$ decreases, cerebral vasoconstriction occurs, with a decrease in CBF. The Pao_2 does not cause so great an effect. The CBF is affected only by severe hypoxemia (less than 50 mm Hg Pao_2).[1]

Viscosity of blood is another factor to consider for adequate CBF. Three factors contribute to blood viscosity: hematocrit, aggregability of erythrocytes, and viscosity of plasma. As the viscosity of blood is decreased (hematocrit decreased), CBF increases.[1,10] A hematocrit of approximately 30% may be ideal for cerebral oxygen delivery.[1]

Body temperature also affects CBF. CBF and the cerebral metabolic rate are decreased with hypothermia. CBF and the cerebral metabolic rate are increased with hyperthermia.[1]

Blood-Brain Barrier

The blood-brain barrier is composed of microvessels and specialized cells. The tight junctions in the endothelial cells provide a barrier to paracellular diffusion of molecules. Only small lipid molecules (less than 400 Da) can be transported by solute transporters from the blood to the brain interstitium. In addition, the blood-brain barrier removes toxins and drugs via efflux transporters.[12] Water, carbon dioxide, oxygen, and lipophilic molecules can cross the blood-brain barrier. Protein molecules and most ions are unable to diffuse.[1]

Brain Injury

Primary brain injury is a pathologic insult to the brain. Examples of primary brain injury include ischemic stroke, hemorrhagic stroke, and traumatic brain injury. The primary brain injury causes an interruption in CBF and therefore cerebral perfusion. Secondary brain injury occurs owing to ischemia, edema, and increased ICP.[6]

Cerebral ischemia results when the delivery of oxygen and glucose to the brain is decreased to the point of interruption of cellular metabolism. If CBF is less than 10 mL/100 g/min, a cascade of events disrupts cellular function. Glutamate, an excitatory amino acid, is released. An influx of calcium and sodium ions into the cell is promoted by the release of glutamate. The increased calcium level may promote the activation of proteases and lipases, which then promote cell membrane injury due to lipid peroxidation and free radical release. The resultant cytotoxic edema causes necrotic cell death, which leads to brain tissue infarction.[1,6]

Cerebral edema is caused by either cytotoxic or vasogenic edema. Cytotoxic edema occurs as a result of the cellular edema described above. Vasogenic edema occurs as a result of the leakage of fluid and solutes into the brain interstitium caused by damage to the blood-brain barrier. Cerebral edema causes increased ICP.[6]

Additional brain injury can occur as a result of reperfusion of ischemic brain tissue. With restoration of cerebral perfusion, oxygen-derived free radicals form. The enzymatic clearance systems that are normally present are exhausted in the ischemic state, thus cell injury occurs as a result of damage by the oxygen-derived free radicals.[6,13]

Injury to the brain can be worsened by cerebral vasospasm, which can cause ischemia and infarction.[6] In cerebral vasospasm, which typically occurs after subarachnoid hemorrhage, the large intracranial arteries respond to the presence of the by-products of clot breakdown by constricting.[14] Oxyhemoglobin is the main by-product of concern in this process.[14,15]

Vasospasm is characterized as either clinical or angiographic. Clinical vasospasm presents with neurologic deficits that mimic ischemic deficits.[15] Cerebral infarction may result owing to decreased CBF with decreased oxygen delivery to the area supplied by the artery in spasm.[14] Angiographic vasospasm is seen with angiographic imaging.[14]

NEUROMONITORING TECHNIQUES

Monitoring ICP and CPP continues to be recognized in the critical care area as a standard of care to provide information relative to brain perfusion and oxygenation for patients with brain injury.[11,16] With the development of several new neuromonitoring techniques, practitioners have an opportunity to positively impact intensive care treatment. Recently developed neuromonitoring techniques include transcranial Doppler (TCD), jugular venous oxygen saturation ($SjvO_2$), partial tissue oxygenation pressure ($PbtO_2$), cerebral microdialysis, near-infrared spectroscopy (NIRS), electrophysiology, and electrocorticography.[17,18]

ICP

ICP can be monitored by using strain gauge technology, either an external strain gauge or a catheter tip strain gauge, or by use of fiber-optic technology. Monitoring devices can be placed in various locations in the brain: ventricular, subarachnoid, subdural, epidural, and parenchymal. The ventricular catheter is the reference standard for monitoring ICP. In addition, the ICP monitoring system that provides the most accuracy and cost-effectiveness is a ventricular catheter attached to an external strain gauge.[16]

The advantage of monitoring ICP is that it is a continuous assessment. The disadvantages are that it requires an invasive procedure with the potential for causing additional brain damage.[17]

CPP

Monitoring the ICP is only a portion of the equation. The CPP is calculated as MAP − ICP. As previously stated, maintaining CPP between 50 and 70 mm Hg has been suggested as the target CPP. However, the optimum CPP to affect positive patient outcomes remains unclear.[7,11]

The advantage of monitoring CPP is that it provides a continuous assessment. The disadvantages are that regional perfusion is not assessed and that CPP is impossible to obtain without an ICP measurement.[17]

TCD

The procedure for performing TCD involves the noninvasive application of sonography to the cranium.[19] The mean CBF velocities of the middle cerebral and intracranial carotid arteries have been used to diagnose cerebral vasospasm. High flow (greater than 200 cm/s) indicates angiographic vasospasm, whereas low flow (less than 120 cm/s) indicates a lesser likelihood of vasospasm.[15]

Because TCD is a noninvasive procedure, it has been suggested to use the pulsatility index (PI) as a reflection of ICP. The PI is calculated by using the CBF velocities (systolic, diastolic, and mean) of the middle cerebral artery. Specifically, the PI is calculated by subtracting the diastolic velocity from the systolic velocity and then dividing the difference by the mean velocity: (systolic CBF velocity − diastolic CBF velocity)/mean CBF velocity. Decreased diastolic CBF velocity (less than 20 cm/s), an increased PI (greater than 1.4), and a peaked waveform indicate decreased CBF.[20]

Although TCD has predictive value for complications of brain injury, such as vasospasm, it has not been shown to be an accurate monitoring tool.[19] Zweifel and colleagues[21] found that using TCD to calculate PI yielded a weak association to ICP and CPP.

The advantage of performing TCD is that it is an indirect assessment (noninvasive) for cerebral perfusion and ICP. The disadvantages are that it is not a continuous assessment, it requires expertise in the performance and reading, and it cannot differentiate vasospasm from hyperemia.[17]

Jugular Venous Oxygenation

Monitoring $SjvO_2$ can provide information concerning cerebral oxygenation and cerebral metabolism.[19] Gupta and colleagues[22] stated in 1999 that monitoring $SvjO_2$ had become widely used to monitor cerebral oxygenation. Typically, the right internal jugular vein has been the choice for retrograde cannulation because it is the dominant internal jugular vein. Continuous monitoring via a fiber-optic catheter or intermittent monitoring via withdrawal of venous blood samples can be accomplished with this method.[19]

$SjvO_2$ directly correlates with cerebral perfusion but indirectly correlates with cerebral oxygen consumption.[17] The value reflects the ratio between CBF and $CMRO_2$. Normal $SjvO_2$ ranges from 55% to 71%.[19] Cerebral ischemia is suggested when the $SjvO_2$ value falls below 55%, which indicates increased oxygen extraction.[18] The values obtained in $SjvO_2$ monitoring, indicating jugular venous desaturation, can be used to make ventilation adjustments when the CPP is decreased.[19]

Even though monitoring $SjvO_2$ is an important tool used to monitor cerebral oxygenation, its benefit to patient outcome remains unclear.[19] The advantage of this method is that it is continuous when the fiber-optic catheter is used. The disadvantages are that it is not continuous if intermittent blood samples are used, the sensors of the fiber-optic catheter have limited stability, the venous cannulation is associated with increased risks, and cerebral venous outflow can be impaired.[17]

Brain Tissue Oxygen Tension

The measurement of brain $PbtO_2$ requires the insertion of invasive fiber-optic monitoring probes into parenchymal tissue.[23] Normal $PbtO_2$ ranges from 25 to 40 mm Hg. A $PbtO_2$ less than 20 mm Hg is considered to be compromised. Brain hypoxia occurs at less than 15 mm Hg.[24]

Placement of the $PbtO_2$ monitoring probe has been a controversial topic. Usually, the probe and the ICP monitor are placed at the same site. This practice limits the choice of optimum location for the best prognostic information.[25] Ponce and colleagues[25] conducted a study in which the placement location of the probe was found to have an effect on the relationship between $PbtO_2$ and long-term neurologic outcome. Instead of placement of the probe in the normal brain only, which had been the typical practice before this study, in a portion of the population studied, the probe was placed in abnormal brain tissue.[25]

On the basis of the placement location of the probe, Ponce and colleagues[25] found that $PbtO_2$ and long-term neurologic outcome are related. Probe placement revealed that the probability for a favorable outcome as the average $PbtO_2$ increases is greater in abnormal brain tissue than in normal brain tissue.[25]

By using the information obtained from carefully monitoring $PbtO_2$, lower mortality rates and better patient outcomes have been obtained than with ICP/CPP monitoring and therapy alone.[24] However, the efficacy of this type of neuromonitoring needs to be validated through larger studies.[26]

PbtO$_2$ monitoring has not been widely accepted in critical care, specifically neuro-intensive care. A study is currently recruiting participants to study whether PbtO$_2$ monitoring improves patient outcomes in the traumatic brain injury population. This study is designed to obtain data for other studies with the overall goal of standardizing treatment modalities in brain tissue oxygenation.[27]

The advantage of PbtO$_2$ monitoring is that it is continuous. The disadvantages are that it provides information only on the brain tissue in which the probe is placed, the probe placement is invasive and can cause additional brain damage, and it is expensive.[17]

Cerebral Microdialysis

Cerebral microdialysis is a monitoring technique that allows for the measurement of changes in substances contained in brain extracellular fluid. Cerebral microdialysis is accomplished by implanting a closed tip catheter into brain parenchyma.[12,17,28] The area of brain that is typically used is the frontal lobe of the nondominant hemisphere.[17,28] Perfusion fluid is pumped between a dialysis membrane and an inner tube. Molecules diffuse across the microdialysis membrane between the brain extracellular fluid and the perfusion fluid. Molecules from the brain extracellular fluid can then be sampled from the perfusion fluid returned from the implanted area.[12]

The substances of particular interest are the markers of metabolism: glucose, lactate, and pyruvate.[12,17] An increased cerebral lactate value characterizes cerebral hypoxia or ischemia.[19] An elevated lactate to pyruvate ratio (lactate:pyruvate), greater than 20 to 25, indicates cerebral ischemia.[19] Experimental models have revealed mitochondrial dysfunction with an elevated lactate:pyruvate ratio, which remains unexplained.[28] Other substances that can be monitored are neurotransmitters, biomarkers for membrane damage and inflammation, and drugs.[12]

The lactate:pyruvate ratio can be used to predict favorable versus unfavorable patient outcome by using 25 as the threshold for unfavorable outcome in patients with traumatic brain injury. Treatment interventions that alter brain chemistry to be used in conjunction with microdialysis have yet to be determined.[28]

The advantages of cerebral microdialysis are that it is not a continuous assessment of cerebral metabolism and that it is an indirect method for assessing cerebral perfusion and oxygenation.[17] The disadvantages are that information is obtained from a specific area of brain and that it requires a surgical procedure that places the patient at an increased risk of brain damage. Also, cerebral microdialysis is expensive.[17] Its characteristic of being discontinuous could be construed to be a disadvantage because the information gathered is intermittent.

NIRS

NIRS monitors cerebral oxygenation through the application of noninvasive optical probes to the patient's forehead.[29] NIRS measures regional cerebral tissue oxygenation saturation (rSO$_2$). The process is based on photon transmission, penetration, and reflection in cerebral tissue and the light-absorbing properties of the chromophores, hemoglobin, and deoxyhemaglobin.[29] Comparison of the wavelengths of oxygenated and deoxygenated hemoglobin can be accomplished through this method.[19,29,30] Oxygen saturation and hemoglobin content in cerebral tissue is measured.[29] The normal value of rSO$_2$ is 60% to 80%.[31]

Various devices have been developed to measure different indices of oxygenation in the brain. The indices include cerebral tissue oxygen saturation, rSO$_2$, and the tissue oxygenation index. Although NIRS has promising potential for use to monitor brain oxygenation, one of the limitations is that extracranial tissue may contaminate the signal.[32]

Adjunctive Neuromonitoring Techniques

Other neuromonitoring techniques include electroencephalograms and electrocorticography. These procedures provide information concerning the electrophysiologic aspect of the brain relative to seizure activity rather than tissue perfusion and oxygenation.[18]

Brain Imaging for Cerebral Perfusion

Although this discussion is focused on bedside neuromonitoring techniques, it is prudent to mention 2 diagnostic procedures used to measure brain tissue perfusion. These procedures can be seen in the literature to measure the effectiveness of bedside neuromonitoring techniques. Both these procedures expose the patient to ionizing radiation and require transport of a critically ill patient, which are potentially dangerous for the patient.

Single-photon emission computed tomography (SPECT) provides cross-sectional images of the brain by using a rotating gamma camera to detect the distribution of an intravenously injected radioactive substance. The radioactive substance typically used is iodine (^{123}I) or technetium (^{99m}Tc). Through the detection of this radioactive substance in the cross-sectional images, a map of brain perfusion can be attained. Even though important information concerning cerebral perfusion is attained through this radiological procedure, it has some negative characteristics. It is expensive, it provides limited anatomic information, and the same information can be obtained more readily through other procedures, such as computed tomography, computed tomography angiography, or perfusion magnetic resonance imaging.[33]

Similar to SPECT, positron emission tomography (PET) uses a gamma-ray detector system that detects emissions of a different radioactive substance. Fludeoxyglucose F 18[33,34] is either inhaled or intravenously injected.[35] Cross-sectional images of the brain capture the concentration of the radioactive substance, which indicates glucose metabolism. A greater uptake of the radioactive substance indicates an increased metabolism of glucose. PET is also expensive, but it provides more anatomic information than does SPECT. The visualization of glucose metabolism provides information concerning cerebral perfusion and overall brain function.[33]

SUMMARY

ICP and CPP remain the mainstays of neuromonitoring because they relate to adequate CBF and brain tissue perfusion and oxygenation. The optimum CPP for maintaining CBF and autoregulation that enhances patient outcome is as yet unknown.[11] The procedure required to attain the readings is invasive and places the patient at risk for complications, such as infection and bleeding.

The procedure for TCD is noninvasive. However, it requires expertise for accurate interpretation.

The Guidelines for the Management of Severe Traumatic Brain Injury state that the monitoring systems that have provided sufficient clinical experience to relate the data collected to patient outcomes are $SjvO_2$ and $PbtO_2$.[36] Yet, both $SjvO_2$ and $PbtO_2$ receive a class III recommendation in the guidelines, which indicates a lack of clinical certainty.[36] Both these techniques place the patient at risk for infection and bleeding because the monitoring devices are placed invasively.

Cerebral microdialysis also places the patient at risk for infection and bleeding because a special catheter must be implanted in brain parenchyma. Questions concerning the utilization of the information obtained and treatment parameters require more research.

NIRS is noninvasive. However, contamination of the signal is problematic and causes concern with accuracy.

More research using randomized controlled trials is needed to determine the most efficient and efficacious bedside neuromonitoring techniques. The ultimate goal is to improve patient outcomes through the development of treatment modalities in response to the information obtained from monitoring brain tissue perfusion and oxygenation.

REFERENCES

1. Butterworth JF IV, Mackey DC, Wasnick JD. Chapter 26. Neurophysiology & anesthesia. In: Butterworth JF IV, Mackey DC, Wasnick JD, editors. Morgan & Mikhail's clinical anesthesiology. 5th edition. New York: McGraw-Hill; 2013. Available at: http://accessmedicine.mhmedical.com/content.aspx?bookid=564& Sectionid=42800558. Accessed February 10, 2014.
2. Ropper AH, Samuels MA. Chapter 34. Cerebrovascular diseases. In: Ropper AH, Samuels MA, editors. Adams and Victor's principles of neurology. 9th edition. New York: McGraw-Hill; 2009. Available at: http://accessmedicine.mhmedical.com/content.aspx?bookid=354&Sectionid=40236347. Accessed February 10, 2014.
3. Barrett KE, Boitano S, Barman SM, et al. Chapter 33. Circulation through special regions. In: Barrett KE, Boitano S, Barman SM, et al, editors. Ganong's review of medical physiology. 24th edition. New York: McGraw-Hill; 2012. Available at: http://accessmedicine.mhmedical.com/content.aspx?bookid=393& Sectionid=39736779. Accessed February 10, 2014.
4. Zuckerbraun BS, Peitzman AB, Billiar TR. Chapter 5. Shock. In: Brunicardi F, Andersen DK, Billiar TR, et al, editors. Schwartz's principles of surgery. 9th edition. New York: McGraw-Hill; 2010. Available at: http://accessmedicine.mhmedical.com/content.aspx?bookid=352&Sectionid=40039746. Accessed January 31, 2014.
5. Cryer PE, Davis SN. Chapter 345. Hypoglycemia. In: Longo DL, Fauci AS, Kasper DL, et al, editors. Harrison's principles of internal medicine. 18th edition. New York: McGraw-Hill; 2012. Available at: http://accessmedicine.mhmedical.com/content.aspx?bookid=331&Sectionid=40727150. Accessed February 10, 2014.
6. Hemphill JC III, Smith WS, Gress DR. Chapter 275. Neurologic critical care, including hypoxic-ischemic encephalopathy, and subarachnoid hemorrhage. In: Longo DL, Fauci AS, Kasper DL, et al, editors. Harrison's principles of internal medicine. 18th edition. New York: McGraw-Hill; 2012. Available at: http://www.accessmedicine.com/content.aspx?aID=9111325. Accessed September 13, 2013.
7. White H, Venkatesh B. Cerebral perfusion pressure in neurotrauma: a review. Anesth Analg 2008;107:979–88.
8. Ropper AH, Samuels MA. Chapter 30. Disturbances of cerebrospinal fluid and its circulation, including hydrocephalus, pseudotumor cerebri, and low-pressure syndromes. In: Ropper AH, Samuels MA, editors. Adams and Victor's principles of neurology. 9th edition. New York: McGraw-Hill; 2009.

Available at: http://www.accessmedicine.com/content.aspx?aID=3635067. Accessed September 16, 2013.

9. Frank JI, Rosengart AJ. Chapter 65. Intracranial pressure: monitoring and management. In: Hall JB, Schmidt GA, Wood LD, editors. Principles of critical care. 3rd edition. New York: McGraw-Hill; 2005. Available at: http://www.accessmedicine.com/content.aspx?aID=2292905. Accessed September 13, 2013.

10. Bor-Seng-Shu E, Kita WS, Figueiredo EG, et al. Cerebral hemodynamics: concepts of clinical importance. Arq Neuropsiquiatr 2012;70:352–6. Available at: http://www.scielo.br/scielo.php?script=sci_arttext&pid=S0004-282X2012000500010&lng=en&nrm=iso. Accessed September 16, 2013.

11. Brain Trauma Foundation, American Association of Neurological Surgeons, Congress of Neurological Surgeons, et al. Guidelines for the management of severe traumatic brain injury. IX Cerebral perfusion thresholds. J Neurotrauma 2007;24:S59–64.

12. Shannon RJ, Carpenter KL, Guilfoyle MR, et al. Cerebral microdialysis in clinical studies of drugs: pharmacokinetic applications. J Pharmacokinet Pharmacodyn 2013;40:343–58.

13. Jan BV, Lowry SF. Chapter 2. Systemic response to injury and metabolic support. In: Brunicardi F, Andersen DK, Billiar TR, et al, editors. Schwartz's principles of surgery. 9th edition. New York: McGraw-Hill; 2010. Available at: http://accessmedicine.mhmedical.com/content.aspx?bookid=352&Sectionid=40039743. Accessed January 22, 2014.

14. Diringer MN, Axelrod Y. Hemodynamic manipulation in the neuro-intensive care unit: cerebral perfusion pressure therapy in head injury and hemodynamic augmentation for cerebral vasospasm. Curr Opin Crit Care 2007;13:156–62.

15. Aiyagari V, Powers WJ, Diringer MN. Chapter 63. Cerebrovascular disease. In: Hall JB, Schmidt GA, Wood LH, editors. Principles of critical care. 3rd edition. New York: McGraw-Hill; 2005. Available at: http://accessmedicine.mhmedical.com/content.aspx?bookid=361&Sectionid=39866433. Accessed January 28, 2014.

16. Brain Trauma Foundation, American Association of Neurological Surgeons, Congress of Neurological Surgeons, et al. Guidelines for the management of severe traumatic brain injury. VII Intracranial pressure monitoring technology. J Neurotrauma 2007;24:S45–54.

17. Stover JF. Actual evidence for neuromonitoring-guided intensive care following severe traumatic brain injury. Swiss Med Wkly 2011;141:w13245.

18. Feyen BF, Sener S, Jorens PG, et al. Neuromonitoring in traumatic brain injury. Minerva Anestesiol 2012;78:949–58.

19. Haddad SH, Arabi YM. Critical care management of severe traumatic brain injury in adults. Scand J Trauma Resusc Emerg Med 2012;20:1–15. Available at: http://www.sjtrem.com/content/20/1/12. Accessed January 15, 2014.

20. Bouzat P, Sala N, Payen JF, et al. Beyond intracranial pressure: optimization of cerebral blood flow, oxygen, and substrate delivery after traumatic brain injury. Ann Intensive Care 2013;3:23. Available at: http://www.annalsofintensivecare.com/content/3/1/23. Accessed January 15, 2014.

21. Zweifel C, Czosnyka M, Carrera E, et al. Reliability of the blood flow velocity pulsatility index for assessment of intracranial and cerebral perfusion pressures in head-injured patients. Neurosurgery 2012;71:853–61.

22. Gupta AK, Hutchinson PJ, Al-Rawi P, et al. Measuring brain tissue oxygenation compared with jugular venous oxygenation saturation for monitoring cerebral oxygenation after traumatic brain injury. Anesth Analg 1999;88:549–53.

23. Rose JC, Neill TA, Hemphill JC. Continuous monitoring of the microcirculation in neurocritical care: an update on brain tissue oxygenation. Curr Opin Crit Care 2006;12:97–102.

24. Spiotta AM, Stiefel MF, Gracia VH, et al. Brain tissue oxygen-directed management and outcome in patients with severe traumatic brain injury. J Neurosurg 2010;113:571–80.

25. Ponce LL, Pillai S, Cruz J, et al. Position of probe determines prognostic information of brain tissue PO2 in severe traumatic brain injury. Neurosurgery 2012;70: 1492–503.

26. Ekbal NJ, Dyson A, Black C, et al. Monitoring tissue perfusion, oxygenation, and metabolism in critically ill patients. Chest 2013;143:1799–808.

27. National Institutes of Health, Health & Human Services. Brain tissue oxygen monitoring in traumatic brain injury (TBI) (BOOST2). Available at: http://www.clinicaltrials.gov/ct2/show/NCT00974259?term=NCT00974259&rank=1. Accessed February 10, 2014.

28. Timofeev I, Carpenter KL, Nortje J, et al. Cerebral extracellular chemistry and outcome following traumatic brain injury: a microdialysis study of 223 patients. Brain 2011;134:484–94.

29. Murkin JM, Arango M. Near-infrared spectroscopy as an index of brain and tissue oxygenation. Br J Anaesth 2009;103:i3–13.

30. Taussky P, O'Neal B, Daugherty WP, et al. Validation of frontal near-infrared spectroscopy as noninvasive bedside monitoring for regional cerebral blood flow in brain-injured patients. Neurosurg Focus 2012;32:1–6.

31. Frost EA. Cerebral oximetry: emerging applications for an established technology. Anesthesiology News 2012. Available at: http://www.anesthesiologynews.com/download/CerebralOximetry_AN0412_WM.pdf. Accessed February 10, 2014.

32. Ghosh A, Elwell C, Smith M. Cerebral near-infrared spectroscopy in adults: a work in progress. Anesth Analg 2012;115:1373–83.

33. Zapadka ME, Bradbury MS, Williams DW III. Chapter 12. Brain and its coverings. In: Chen MM, Pope TL, Ott DJ, editors. Basic radiology. 2nd edition. New York: McGraw-Hill; 2011. Available at: http://accessmedicine.mhmedical.com/content.aspx?bookid=360&Sectionid=39669022. Accessed February 7, 2014.

34. Dillon WP. Chapter 368. Neuroimaging in neurologic disorders. In: Longo DL, Fauci AS, Kasper DL, et al, editors. Harrison's principles of internal medicine. 18th edition. New York: McGraw-Hill; 2012. Available at: http://accessmedicine.mhmedical.com/content.aspx?bookid=331&Sectionid=40727180. Accessed February 9, 2014.

35. Waxman SG. Chapter 22. Imaging of the brain. In: Waxman SG, editor. Clinical neuroanatomy. 27th edition. New York: McGraw-Hill; 2013. Available at: http://accessmedicine.mhmedical.com/content.aspx?bookid=673&Sectionid=45395988. Accessed February 9, 2014.

36. Brain Trauma Foundation, American Association of Neurological Surgeons, Congress of Neurological Surgeons, et al. Guidelines for the management of severe traumatic brain injury. X Brain oxygen monitoring and thresholds. J Neurotrauma 2007;24:S65–70.

Microcirculatory Alterations in Shock States

Shannan K. Hamlin, PhD, RN, ACNP-BC, AGACNP-BC, CCRN[a,*],
C. Lee Parmley, MD, JD, MMHC[b,c], Sandra K. Hanneman, PhD, RN[d]

KEYWORDS

- Microcirculation • Oxygen transport • Oxygen utilization • Oxygen extraction
- Blood flow • Hypovolemic shock • Cardiogenic shock • Septic shock

KEY POINTS

- In health, functional components of the microcirculation provide oxygen and nutrients and remove waste products from the tissue beds of the body's organs.
- Shock states overwhelmingly stress functional capacity of the microcirculation, resulting in microcirculatory failure.
- In septic shock, there is abundant evidence that inflammatory mediators cause or contribute to hemodynamic instability.
- In nonseptic shock states, the microcirculation is better able to compensate for alterations in vascular resistance, cardiac output (CO), and blood pressure.
- Autoregulation at the arteriolar level and the endothelium and erythrocyte at the cellular level maintain oxygen diffusion gradients sufficient to support aerobic metabolism.
- In comparison with septic shock, hypovolemic and cardiogenic shock states are not challenged with the additional burden of infection and its consequential effects on the microcirculation.
- Global hemodynamic and oxygen delivery ($\dot{D}O_2$) parameters are appropriate for assessing, monitoring, and guiding therapy in hypovolemic and cardiogenic shock but, alone, are inadequate for septic shock.

Funding Sources: None.
Conflict of Interest: None.
[a] Nursing Research and Evidence-Based Practice, Houston Methodist Hospital, MGJ 11-017, Houston, TX 77030, USA; [b] Vanderbilt University Hospital, 1211 21st Avenue South, S3408 MCN, Nashville, TN 37212, USA; [c] Department of Anesthesiology, Division of Critical Care, Vanderbilt University School of Medicine, 1211 21st Avenue South, S3408 MCN, Nashville, TN 37212, USA; [d] Center for Nursing Research, University of Texas Health Science Center at Houston School of Nursing, Room #594, 6901 Bertner Avenue, Houston, TX 77030, USA
* Corresponding author.
E-mail address: SHamlin@HoustonMethodist.org

INTRODUCTION

A functional microcirculation is essential for adequate tissue perfusion. In critically ill patients, microvascular function frequently is altered, which can lead to cellular hypoxia, organ dysfunction, and poor outcomes.[1] All shock profiles have some degree of microvascular dysfunction, but a distressed microcirculation is the hallmark of septic shock. Microvascular dysfunction impairs tissue oxygenation during sepsis, and prolonged microvascular alterations are associated with higher rates of multiple organ dysfunction syndrome (MODS) and mortality.[2] Monitoring of the microcirculation is beyond the capabilities of technology routinely available at the bedside, but new monitoring methods are being developed, refined, and tested.

The macrocirculation (ie, the arteries and veins) is more readily and routinely monitored than the microcirculation. Global measures of hemodynamic and oxygen transport, such as CO, mean arterial pressure (MAP), $\dot{D}O_2$, oxygen consumption ($\dot{V}O_2$), and systemic vascular resistance (SVR), are used to evaluate the macrocirculation. These measures may be sufficient for most patients with hypovolemic and cardiogenic shock who do not have profound hypotension; however, they are insufficient for monitoring the adequacy of microvascular blood flow in patients with septic shock,[3] and the outcome is related to how quickly the microvasculature recovers.[4,5]

In this article, the authors review the microcirculatory alterations found in hypovolemic, cardiogenic, and septic shock. The general physiologic function of the microcirculation in the nonseptic shock states serves as the foundation for an in-depth development of the more complex disruptions that occur in septic shock.

GENERAL PRINCIPLES OF MICROVASCULAR FUNCTION

Factors that influence microvascular function include oxygen transport mechanisms and the cell's endothelium. Capillary blood flow (convective transport) and capillary density (diffusive transport)[2] ultimately determine tissue perfusion.[6] Convective and diffusive oxygen transport mechanisms are altered in septic shock, which affects both $\dot{D}O_2$ and tissue perfusion.

Convective and Diffusive Oxygen Transport

Convective oxygen transport (bulk transport of oxygen by blood over long distances) is determined by microvascular blood oxygen content and flow.[3] Arterioles, the resistance vessels, predominately control interorgan and intraorgan blood flow by vasoregulation. Oxygen is transported to tissues from the capillary bed by diffusive oxygen transport (movement of oxygen from the microcirculation to the cell's mitochondria). The adequacy of tissue oxygenation depends on microvascular $\dot{D}O_2$, the critical oxygen diffusion distance (eg, the maximum distance the mitochondria can be away from an oxygen source), and intercapillary distance.[7] A reduction in capillary density increases the diffusion distance for oxygen,[8] and anaerobic metabolism will occur when a critical point in diffusion distance is reached.[3]

Endothelium and Nitric Oxide

The endothelium is a highly specialized tissue that lines the microvascular system.[9] An intact endothelium is crucial to overall microcirculatory function along with nitric oxide (NO), also known as endothelial relaxing factor. To maintain vascular homeostasis and organ perfusion under physiologic conditions,[10–12] endothelial cells sense blood-borne signals and changes in hemodynamic forces based on local shear stress and membrane receptor mechanisms. The endothelial luminal surface is covered by a layer of glycocalyx, which contributes to vascular barrier competence and facilitates red blood cell (RBC) flow by limiting adhesion of white blood cells (WBCs) and platelets to the endothelial surface.[2,12,13] The endothelium modulates immune responses and regulates coagulation and inflammatory and vasoactive agents in the blood.[14] Through cell-to-cell signaling,[15] the capillary endothelium communicates with upstream arterioles to autoregulate vasomotor tone, primarily through local release of vasodilators such as NO, and recruit microvessels to increase capillary blood flow.

NO is a highly reactive free radical formed from oxidation of L-arginine.[16] The many physiologic effects of NO include potent vasodilation to maintain vascular tone[12] and modulation of hemorheologic behavior[11] to increase RBC deformability and reduce leukocyte and platelet adhesion and platelet aggregation.[17–19] Because NO indirectly lowers perfusion pressure, NO inhibition has been studied extensively with considerable research focused on the L-arginine analogues (eg, N^G-monomethyl-L-arginine [L-NMMA] and N-nitro-L-arginine methyl ester [L-NAME]), which competitively and directly inhibit NO synthase.[20] Studies in both human and animal models have shown considerable increases in MAP and SVR with NO inhibition.[21–26] However, a phase III clinical trial using nonspecific NO synthase inhibition was discontinued early because of increased mortality from progressive cardiac failure, despite improvement in MAP and CO.[20,27]

Blood and Blood Flow

Capillary blood flow is determined by the driving pressure, arterial tone, and rheologic factors such as vessel geometry and RBC deformability.[7,28] The mobile RBC modulates local vascular tone by sensing hypoxic stimuli in the microvasculature and releasing adenosine 5'-triphosphate (ATP).[29,30] ATP causes endothelium-dependent vasorelaxation.[31] Within the vasculature, intraluminal ATP induces vasodilation by binding to purinergic receptors via endothelial cells along the vessels upstream from the capillary in an effort to augment local tissue perfusion by matching oxygen supply to demand.[30] It seems that NO plays a role in the ATP-vasodilation process but this has not been fully elucidated.[32] From the current evidence, the RBC itself has a role in determining oxygen supply to tissues.[29]

Vasodilation of precapillary arterioles opens closed capillaries, thereby recruiting an increased number to carry the same volume of blood flow.[10] Vasodilation increases mean capillary transit time, and oxygen more rapidly traverses the capillary, producing an increased Po_2 gradient and tissue oxygen utilization. This capillary recruitment reduces intercapillary and oxygen diffusion distance, both of which are important components of optimizing diffusive oxygen transport.[10] Indeed, ATP introduced into the vessel lumen can increase the arteriolar diameter up to 8% and capillary RBC supply by up to 6 cells per second, which is immediately followed by a 2- to 3-mm Hg increase in Po_2.[33]

In physiologic conditions, organ blood flow is in accordance with metabolic requirements so that each organ receives a fraction of whole-body $\dot{D}o_2$.[14] Minor alterations in the redistribution of blood flow, as happens when organs that are able to increase the oxygen extraction ratio (O_2ER) receive a smaller fraction of flow, significantly affect whole-body critical $\dot{D}o_2$ by forcing $\dot{V}o_2$ to become supply dependent.[14]

MICROCIRCULATION ALTERATIONS IN HYPOVOLEMIC SHOCK

Microcirculatory alterations in hypovolemic shock may be small, as the microvasculature is still able to function and regulate microvascular perfusion.[34] If the blood pressure is dramatically decreased, there is a decrease in functional capillary density in patients with hypovolemic shock, but this change recovers quickly with hemodynamic restoration.[35]

Using a mouse model, Nakajima and colleagues[36] compared microvascular perfusion in hemorrhagic hypovolemic shock with that in septic shock at comparable levels of hypotension.[36] Compared with the septic shock model, the researchers found a lower percentage of nonperfused capillaries, preserved RBC velocity, and appropriate regulation of microvascular perfusion in the subjects with hypovolemic shock.

In hypovolemic shock, microvascular alterations are not completely disassociated from global measures of oxygen transport, which is true in cardiogenic shock as well,[37] which is discussed later. Few studies have been conducted evaluating the impact of hypovolemic shock on the microcirculation, and the standard of care remains volume replacement therapy to improve organ perfusion and thereby organ function.[35]

MICROCIRCULATION ALTERATIONS IN CARDIOGENIC SHOCK

Cardiogenic shock is characterized by inadequate organ perfusion from cardiac dysfunction, which causes decreased CO despite adequate intravascular volume.[37] In severe cardiogenic shock, microvascular perfusion is altered even when normal values of global hemodynamic parameters are restored.[38] De Backer and colleagues[39] showed, in patients with cardiogenic shock, a decrease in the number of perfused capillaries within 48 hours of the onset of acute heart failure wherein the severity of heart failure was associated with patient mortality.

Although the exact microvascular disturbance remains unclear in cardiogenic shock, observations of decreased vessel density have prompted clinicians to consider specific treatment strategies, including pharmacologic interventions and mechanical assist devices, that would lead to improvement in microcirculatory perfusion.[40] Patients who were hemodynamically stable and ready for removal of an intraaortic balloon pump (IABP) had increased microcirculatory flow in small vessels after removal of the IABP.[39] This finding suggests that, in hemodynamically recovered patients, (1) IABP may impair microcirculatory perfusion and clinicians should be vigilant about its timely removal and (2) global hemodynamic parameters are insufficiently sensitive for assessing the microcirculation in patients with cardiogenic shock.[40]

MICROVASCULAR ALTERATIONS IN SEPTIC SHOCK

Impaired microcirculatory blood flow in sepsis likely plays a major role in progression to septic shock.[3] Sepsis represents a constellation of progressive clinical manifestations launched by an infectious insult that serves as a catalyst for systemic inflammatory response syndrome. Septic shock, the most devastating phase of the sepsis continuum, is a state of acute circulatory failure[41]; it is associated with profound hemodynamic alterations, including persistent hypotension, hypovolemia, decreased vascular tone, and myocardial depression. MODS results from such alterations.[41,42]

Microvascular injury may be the key event that leads to MODS.[43] The septic process targets adversely almost every aspect of microvascular circulation[44]: (1) endothelial cell injury[45]; (2) decreased capillary density with increased diffusion distance[46]; (3) heterogeneity (maldistribution) of blood flow and perfusion, independent of perfusion pressure[5]; (4) pathologic shunting of oxygenated blood[47]; and (5) impaired cellular oxygen utilization.[3,46] A combination of inflammatory and procoagulation-mediated[7,48] factors are responsible for microvascular damage in septic shock. These factors affect vascular autoregulation and the rheologic properties[49] of blood, leading to sluggish blood flow in the microcirculation.[1,47]

Endothelial Dysfunction

In septic shock, release of vasoactive substances and cytokines from the endothelium alters the balance between systemic and local vascular controls and results in overall vasodilation.[50] Widespread, unregulated vasoparalysis stems from endothelial and smooth muscle damage and excess NO release generated by the inflammatory response.[43] Many experts think sepsis-induced endothelial injury is the genesis of microvascular dysfunction in septic shock, leading to alterations in organ perfusion and subsequent organ failure (**Fig. 1**).[6,45,51–54]

The endothelial dysfunction observed in sepsis affects vascular responsiveness, $\dot{D}O_2$, and oxygen extraction.[10,52] Inflammatory cytokines increase the expression of adhesion molecules that lead to leukocyte and platelet adhesion to the endothelial surface.[2,51,55] The endothelial glycocalyx layer undergoes degradation,[56] the severity of which is associated with reduced functional capillary density (**Fig. 2**)[57] and increased mortality.[58]

Leukocyte and platelet adherence to the endothelial wall further activates the coagulation and inflammatory cascades, thereby further reducing blood flow. The damaged endothelium results in disordered signaling of precapillary arteriolar regulation, which is necessary for precise control of microvascular perfusion.[59] In a septic

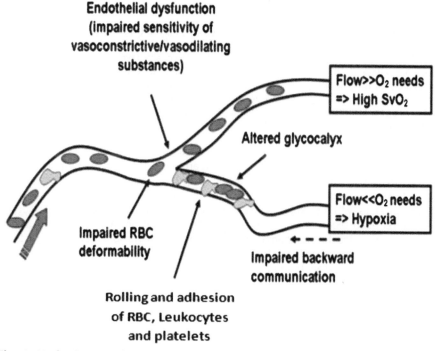

Endothelial dysfunction (impaired sensitivity of vasoconstrictive/vasodilating substances)

Flow>>O$_2$ needs => High SvO$_2$

Altered glycocalyx

Flow<<O$_2$ needs => Hypoxia

Impaired RBC deformability

Impaired backward communication

Rolling and adhesion of RBC, Leukocytes and platelets

Fig. 1. Mechanisms involved in microvascular alterations in septic shock. Endothelial dysfunction results in (1) impaired sensitivity to vasoactive substances; (2) rolling and adhesion of red blood cells (RBC), white blood cells, and platelets; and (3) destruction of the glycocalyx layer. Impaired RBC deformability and backward communication to arterioles signaling reduced blood flow and hypoxia also occur. SVO$_2$, mixed venous oxyhemoglobin saturation. (*From* De Backer D, Donadello K, Taccone FS, et al. Microcirculatory alterations: Potential mechanisms and implications for therapy. Ann Intensive Care 2011;1(1):27; with permission.)

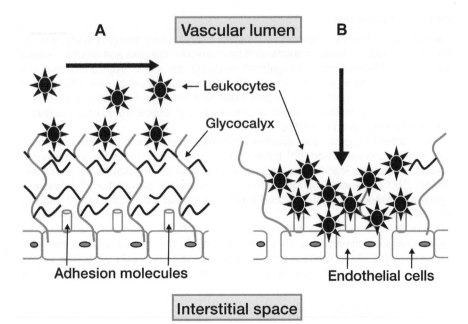

Fig. 2. The intact and degraded endothelial glycocalyx layer. (*A*) An intact glycocalyx layer with nonactivated leukocytes flowing freely in the vessel without contacting the endothelial adhesion molecules. (*B*) Schema of a degraded glycocalyx layer as nonactivated leukocytes are allowed to connect with the exposed and activated endothelial adhesion molecules, causing leukocyte activation, adhesion, migration, and compromised blood flow. (*From* Chappell D, Westphal M, Jacob M. The impact of the glycocalyx on microcirculatory oxygen distribution in critical illness. Curr Opin Anaesthesiol 2009;22(2):158; with permission.)

mouse model, Tyml and colleagues[60] showed that impaired signaling rates in microvessels 500 μm apart resulted in compromised arteriolar responsiveness and conduction levels. The range of arteriovenous path length (ie, vasculature architecture) for signal transduction is 450 to 2077 μm[61]; conductions limited to less than 500 μm would correlate with a sizable decrease in the rate of signal conduction.[32] In conditions of reduced blood flow or hypoxemia, the endothelium normally would signal upstream arterioles to vasoconstrict, increasing the perfusion pressure and thus allowing more oxygen-rich blood to enter the capillary. Endothelial dysfunction impairs this regulation of capillary blood flow.[51]

Nitric Oxide and the Microcirculation

NO is the key molecule in vascular autoregulation.[62] In septic shock, inflammatory cytokines (eg, tumor necrosis factor-α, interleukin-1) and lipopolysaccharide stimulate overproduction of NO,[63,64] a factor in refractory hypotension.[7] The heterogeneous upregulation of inducible NO synthase (iNOS) between and within organ tissues[65] results in a pathologic shunting of flow[66] because tissue areas lacking iNOS have less NO-induced vasodilation and, therefore, experience decreased blood flow and organ perfusion.[6] A state of heterogeneity in tissue perfusion is created[67,68] whereby there is a relative deficiency of NO in some tissues and organs despite a total body excess of NO; this heterogeneity causes pathologic shunting of oxygenated blood away from hypoxic tissues where it is most needed.[69]

Blood Alterations

An important component of sepsis pathology is the attenuation of microvascular cell-to-cell conduction, which affects pathways for vasodilation signals and arteriolar responsiveness.[60] Using the communication ratio, 500 μm upstream, (CR_{500}) as an index for conducted response, Lidington and colleagues[59] reported that sepsis significantly reduced the CR_{500} from 0.75 to 0.20, which had an adverse impact on the control of blood flow. The study findings highlight both the complexity and magnitude of direct and indirect microvascular alterations in septic shock, not to mention the alterations in the blood components themselves.

Sepsis induces intrinsic changes in RBCs,[2] leukocytes, and platelets. The RBC becomes less deformable, making it difficult to traverse the smaller capillary bed.[70] In addition, RBCs are slower to recover their shape and have an increased propensity to aggregate[64] and adhere to the endothelial wall.[71] With an increase in RBC aggregation comes slowing of capillary blood flow, as the blood is more viscous with a tendency to drag, further reducing tissue perfusion.[49] A reduced luminal cross section from aggregation and adherence reduces mean RBC velocity and often makes it impossible for circulating RBCs and leukocytes to pass through the smaller capillary, especially when perfusion pressures are low.[72] The RBC becomes rigid and unshrinkable as viscosity increases and often occludes small capillary vessels.[35]

Similarly, increased leukocyte[73] and platelet[74] adherence to the endothelial wall further disturbs capillary blood flow. Platelet-endothelial adherence occurs within 1 hour of an infectious insult, followed by a surge in leukocyte adherence 3 to 5 hours later; a decrease in microcirculatory perfusion occurs in as little as 3 hours from the initial insult.[55] Secor and colleagues[74] reported a 28% drop in platelet count related to endothelial adhesion in their septic animal model, which corresponded with up to 40% plugging of the capillary bed. A 30% drop in platelet count is an independent predictor of death in critically ill patients.[75]

Blood Flow Alterations

Using an ovine sepsis model, Di Giantomasso and colleagues[76] reported the development of organ dysfunction despite a marked increase in blood flow to the heart, gut, and kidney. This finding suggests that global ischemia may not be the principal pathologic mechanism of vital organ dysfunction.[76] One explanation for organ hypoperfusion, despite an increase in macrocirculation blood flow, may be regional areas of impaired perfusion.

As blood leaves the arterioles, reduced capillary density leads to a reduced surface area available for $\dot{D}O_2$. The cause for this reduced capillary density is multifactorial, including (1) capillary occlusion from circulating RBCs; (2) entrapment of less deformable leukocytes; (3) disseminated intravascular coagulation (DIC), causing cells to aggregate; (4) and capillary endothelial swelling, which reduces luminal size of the capillary and causes entrapment of circulating cells.[43,77] These factors specifically are of concern in sepsis.

Studies have shown increased microvascular heterogeneity during sepsis, with evidence of capillary flow cessation (stopped flow).[46,78,79] The consequences of capillaries with stopped flow, in addition to regional tissue ischemia, include loss of functional capillary density with the attendant increase in oxygen diffusion distance, making it more difficult to oxygenate the remote areas.[7]

Diffusive Oxygen Transport Alterations

Septic shock is characterized by increased stopped-flow capillaries,[67] decreased RBC flow velocity,[46] increased heterogeneity of flow,[80] and low functional capillary density.[52,68] The strongest predictor of outcome is the number of perfused small vessels.[5] Heterogeneity of flow is a critical alteration because of its association with heterogeneity of oxygenation and oxygen extraction.[42] As the number of stopped-flow capillaries increases with decreased capillary density, microvascular perfusion is significantly impaired.[51,67] De Backer and colleagues[79] found that the number of perfused vessels is significantly reduced in septic shock and these alterations are more severe in nonsurvivors than survivors.

Alteration in Oxygen Utilization—Dysoxia

Even with normal macrocirculation parameters,[42] heterogeneous tissue perfusion is associated with heterogeneity in oxygenation[81] and oxygen extraction.[68,80,82–84] These microvascular alterations contribute to both tissue hypoxia and mitochondrial dysfunction.[7]

Numerous animal[67,80] and human studies[85,86] have demonstrated an increase in capillary oxygen extraction as the number of stopped-flow capillaries increase, clearly indicating that the septic microcirculation is unable to regulate flow to regions of higher oxygen demand,[51] which suggests that heterogeneous tissue oxygenation is the result of impaired oxygen extraction linked with heterogeneity of blood flow.[42,68,82–84] Under such conditions, some capillary beds have increased blood flow beyond their metabolic needs and others have reduced blood flow less than their needs.[51] When the critical O_2ER is reached, the cells switch from aerobic to anaerobic metabolism.[84] In short, microvascular dysfunction leads to impaired oxygen extraction in septic shock.[51]

Moreover, there are significant variations in metabolic rate across the spectrum of sepsis presentations. In an observational study comparing basal metabolic rates in healthy individuals and septic patients, sepsis was associated with a 30% increase in basal metabolic rate more than normal. When comparing different septic states, septic shock had the least increase in metabolic rate ($+2 \pm 24\%$) compared with severe sepsis ($+24 \pm 12\%$) and sepsis ($+55 \pm 14\%$).[87] The variation in metabolic rate may be related to oxygen utilization at the mitochondrial level. ATP production from mitochondrial oxidative phosphorylation accounts for more than 90% of $\dot{V}O_2$, and NO overproduction is known to inhibit oxidative phosphorylation.[88] NO overproduction has been linked to mitochondrial dysfunction and decreased ATP concentrations in muscle tissue of septic patients.[88] Both tissue hypoxia and mitochondrial dysfunction are the result of microvascular dysfunction.[7]

The tissue dysoxia of sepsis is thought to stem from inefficient matching of oxygen supply to oxygen demand from vascular dysregulation, both vasoconstriction and dilation. This condition results in impaired oxygen extraction capability, forcing tissue $\dot{V}O_2$ to be supply dependent in some tissue beds.[7,82,84,89] In the setting of increased $\dot{D}O_2$ and $\dot{V}O_2$ in sepsis, alterations in mitochondrial respiration cause reduced oxygen extraction and tissue oxygen debt.[7,14] $\dot{V}O_2$ is a measure of global tissue oxygen use, and a normal value may give the false impression that all tissue beds are adequately extracting oxygen when, in fact, $\dot{V}O_2$ is impaired regionally.

Data on the critical issue of inefficient oxygen use in septic shock are conflicting. It may be caused by impaired mitochondrial respiration, whereby reduced O_2ER is a result of decreased oxygen utilization,[90] or maldistribution of blood flow from microvascular injury and vascular dysregulation, which undersupplies some capillary beds while oversupplying others.[80] A study of stopped-flow capillaries relative to capillary density and intercapillary distance strongly suggests that tissues that receive adequate $\dot{D}O_2$ are capable of extracting oxygen; therefore, functional mitochondrial injury may not exist.[7,80] On the other hand, findings from studies seeking to maximize

$\dot{D}O_2$ to supranormal levels found supranormal values failed to improve tissue oxygenation, suggesting impaired mitochondrial function.[91,92] Although there is ample evidence and theory in pathophysiology to support involvement of both blood flow maldistribution and mitochondrial dysfunction factors, in general, data support the theory that in early-stage sepsis, oxygen transport is compromised by maldistribution of $\dot{D}O_2$ and that heterogeneous tissue oxygenation exists.

CONCLUSIONS AND IMPLICATIONS

In health, functional components of the microcirculation provide oxygen and nutrients and remove waste products from the tissue beds of the body's organs. Shock states overwhelmingly stress functional capacity of the microcirculation, resulting in microcirculatory failure. In septic shock, there is abundant evidence that inflammatory mediators cause or contribute to hemodynamic instability.

In nonseptic shock states, the microcirculation is better able to compensate for alterations in vascular resistance, CO, and blood pressure. Autoregulation at the arteriolar level and the endothelium and erythrocyte at the cellular level maintain oxygen diffusion gradients sufficient to support aerobic metabolism. In comparison with septic shock, hypovolemic and cardiogenic shock states are not challenged with the additional burden of infection and its consequential effects on the microcirculation. Therefore, global hemodynamic and $\dot{D}O_2$ parameters are appropriate for assessing, monitoring, and guiding therapy.

In septic shock, the complex microcirculatory alterations have not been fully elucidated. Strong evidence exists that microvascular alterations cause MODS, and patients have better outcomes when the microvasculature recovers early. The focus is expected to remain on restoring microvasculature function by targeting multiple pathways and on developing new technologies that allow bedside monitoring of the microcirculation.

One such technology is sidestream dark-field (SDF) imaging, wherein a video microscope illuminates tissue with green wavelength light emitting diodes. Hemoglobin absorption of the green light provides images of circulating RBCs.[93] Researchers have used SDF imaging of sublingual microcirculation density and flow to compare the effects of leukocyte-depleted and non-leukocyte-depleted blood transfusions on microcirculatory convective flow of patients in various stages of the sepsis continuum.[94] Others[53] have used SDF imaging to study the relation between early treatment in sepsis and MODS. At present, this technique requires direct probe contact with the tissue (eg, sublingual mucosa); thus, the observations may reflect local or regional microcirculatory function that is unrepresentative of other organ tissues. Nonetheless, continued development of such technologies and future development of imaging techniques that do not require direct contact with tissue hold promise for better understanding, assessment, and treatment of microvasculature dysfunction that improves outcomes of patients, particularly those with septic shock.

REFERENCES

1. De Backer D, Donadello K, Favory R. Link between coagulation abnormalities and microcirculatory dysfunction in critically ill patients. Curr Opin Anaesthesiol 2009;22(2):150–4.
2. De Backer D, Donadello K, Taccone FS, et al. Microcirculatory alterations: potential mechanisms and implications for therapy. Ann Intensive Care 2011;1(1):27.
3. Trzeciak S, Rivers EP. Clinical manifestations of disordered microcirculatory perfusion in severe sepsis. Crit Care 2005;9(Suppl 4):S20–6.

4. Sakr Y, Dubois MJ, De Backer D, et al. Persistent microcirculatory alterations are associated with organ failure and death in patients with septic shock. Crit Care Med 2004;32(9):1825–31.

5. De Backer D, Donadello K, Sakr Y, et al. Microcirculatory alterations in patients with severe sepsis: impact of time of assessment and relationship with outcome. Crit Care Med 2013;41(3):791–9.

6. Ince C. The microcirculation is the motor of sepsis. Crit Care 2005;9(Suppl 4): S13–9.

7. Bateman RM, Sharpe MD, Ellis CG. Bench-to-bedside review: microvascular dysfunction in sepsis-hemodynamics, oxygen transport, and nitric oxide. Crit Care 2003;7(5):359–73.

8. Bateman RM, Tokunaga C, Kareco T, et al. Myocardial hypoxia-inducible HIF-1alpha, VEGF, and GLUT1 gene expression is associated with microvascular and ICAM-1 heterogeneity during endotoxemia. Am J Physiol Heart Circ Physiol 2007;293(1):H448–56.

9. Spronk PE, Zandstra DF, Ince C. Bench-to-bedside review: sepsis is a disease of the microcirculation. Crit Care 2004;8(6):462–8.

10. Vallet B. Endothelial cell dysfunction and abnormal tissue perfusion. Crit Care Med 2002;30(Suppl 5):S229–34.

11. Celermajer DS. Endothelial dysfunction: does it matter? Is it reversible? J Am Coll Cardiol 1997;30(2):325–33.

12. Gori T, Forconi S. Endothelium and hemorheology. In: Baskurt OK, Hardeman MR, Rampling MW, et al, editors. Handbook of hemorheology and hemodynamics. (WA): IOS Press; 2007. p. 339–50.

13. Chappell D, Westphal M, Jacob M. The impact of the glycocalyx on microcirculatory oxygen distribution in critical illness. Curr Opin Anaesthesiol 2009;22(2):155–62.

14. Vallet B. Vascular reactivity and tissue oxygenation. Intensive Care Med 1998; 24(1):3–11.

15. Hungerford JE, Sessa WC, Segal SS. Vasomotor control in arterioles of the mouse cremaster muscle. FASEB J 2000;14(1):197–207.

16. Alderton WK, Cooper CE, Knowles RG. Nitric oxide synthases: structure, function and inhibition. Biochem J 2001;357(Pt 3):593–615.

17. Radomski MW, Vallance P, Whitley G, et al. Platelet adhesion to human vascular endothelium is modulated by constitutive and cytokine induced nitric oxide. Cardiovasc Res 1993;27(7):1380–2.

18. Naseem KM. The role of nitric oxide in cardiovascular diseases. Mol Aspects Med 2005;26(1–2):33–65.

19. Godin C, Caprani A, Dufaux J, et al. Interactions between neutrophils and endothelial cells. J Cell Sci 1993;106(Pt 2):441–51.

20. Finney SJ, Evans TW. Pathophysiology of sepsis: the role of nitric oxide. In: Vincent JL, Carlet J, Opal S, editors. The sepsis text. Boston: Kluwer Academic Publishers; 2002. p. 211–29.

21. Avontuur JA, Tutein Nolthenius RP, van Bodegom JW, et al. Prolonged inhibition of nitric oxide synthesis in severe septic shock: a clinical study. Crit Care Med 1998;26(4):660–7.

22. Lorente JA, Landin L, De Pablo R, et al. L-arginine pathway in the sepsis syndrome. Crit Care Med 1993;21(9):1287–95.

23. Petros A, Lamb G, Leone A, et al. Effects of a nitric oxide synthase inhibitor in humans with septic shock. Cardiovasc Res 1994;28(1):34–9.

24. Petros A, Bennett D, Vallance P. Effect of nitric oxide synthase inhibitors on hypotension in patients with septic shock. Lancet 1991;338(8782–8783):1557–8.

25. Yang S, Cioffi WG, Bland KI, et al. Differential alterations in systemic and regional oxygen delivery and consumption during the early and late stages of sepsis. J Trauma 1999;47(4):706–12.

26. Zhang H, Rogiers P, Smail N, et al. Effects of nitric oxide on blood flow distribution and O2 extraction capabilities during endotoxic shock. J Appl Phys 1997; 83(4):1164–73.

27. Broccard A, Hurni JM, Eckert P, et al. Tissue oxygenation and hemodynamic response to NO synthase inhibition in septic shock. Shock 2000;14:35–40.

28. den Uil CA, Klijn E, Lagrand WK, et al. The microcirculation in health and critical disease. Prog Cardiovasc Dis 2008;51(2):161–70.

29. Dietrich HH, Ellsworth ML, Sprague RS, et al. Red blood cell regulation of microvascular tone through adenosine triphosphate. Am J Physiol Heart Circ Physiol 2000;278(4):H1294–8.

30. Sprague RS, Bowles EA, Achilleus D, et al. Erythrocytes as controllers of perfusion distribution in the microvasculature of skeletal muscle. Acta Physiol (Oxf) 2011;202(3):285–92.

31. Burnstock G, Kennedy C. A dual function for adenosine 5'-triphosphate in the regulation of vascular tone. Excitatory cotransmitter with noradrenaline from perivascular nerves and locally released inhibitory intravascular agent. Circ Res 1986;58(3):319–30.

32. Ellsworth ML. The red blood cell as an oxygen sensor: what is the evidence? Acta Physiol Scand 2000;168(4):551–9.

33. Collins DM, McCullough WT, Ellsworth ML. Conducted vascular responses: communication across the capillary bed. Microvasc Res 1998;56(1):43–53.

34. Ellis CG, Jagger J, Sharpe M. The microcirculation as a functional system. Crit Care 2005;9(Suppl 4):S3–8.

35. Donati A, Domizi R, Damiani E, et al. From macrohemodynamic to the microcirculation. Crit Care Res Pract 2013;2013:892710.

36. Nakajima Y, Baudry N, Duranteau J, et al. Microcirculation in intestinal villi: a comparison between hemorrhagic and endotoxin shock. Am J Respir Crit Care Med 2001;164(8 Pt 1):1526–30.

37. Ashruf JF, Bruining HA, Ince C. New insights into the pathophysiology of cardiogenic shock: the role of the microcirculation. Curr Opin Crit Care 2013;19(5):381–6.

38. Harrois A, Dupic L, Duranteau J. Targeting the microcirculation in resuscitation of acutely unwell patients. Curr Opin Crit Care 2011;17(3):303–7.

39. Munsterman LD, Elbers PW, Ozdemir A, et al. Withdrawing intra-aortic balloon pump support paradoxically improves microvascular flow. Crit Care 2010; 14(4):R161.

40. Jung C, Lauten A, Ferrari M. Microcirculation in cardiogenic shock: from scientific bystander to therapy target. Crit Care 2010;14(5):193.

41. Levy B, Mansart A, Bollaert PE, et al. Effects of epinephrine and norepinephrine on hemodynamics, oxidative metabolism, and organ energetics in endotoxemic rats. Intensive Care Med 2003;29(2):292–300.

42. De Backer D, Orbegozo Cortes D, Donadello K, et al. Pathophysiology of microcirculatory dysfunction and the pathogenesis of septic shock. Virulence 2013; 5(1):73–9.

43. Sielenkamper AW, Kvietys P, Sibbald W. Microvascular alterations in sepsis. In: Vincent JL, Carlet J, Opal S, editors. The sepsis text. Boston: Kluwer Academic Publishers; 2002. p. 247–70.

44. Ince C. Microcirculation in distress: a new resuscitation end point? Crit Care Med 2004;32(9):1963–4.

45. Aird WC. The role of the endothelium in severe sepsis and multiple organ dysfunction syndrome. Blood 2003;101(10):3765–77.
46. Edul VS, Enrico C, Laviolle B, et al. Quantitative assessment of the microcirculation in healthy volunteers and in patients with septic shock. Crit Care Med 2012;40(5):1443–8.
47. Ince C, Sinaasappel M. Microcirculatory oxygenation and shunting in sepsis and shock. Crit Care Med 1999;27(7):1369–77.
48. Levi M, van der Poll T, Buller HR. Bidirectional relation between inflammation and coagulation. Circulation 2004;109(22):2698–704.
49. Piagnerelli M, Boudjeltia KZ, Vanhaeverbeek M, et al. Red blood cell rheology in sepsis. Intensive Care Med 2003;29(7):1052–61.
50. Hinshaw LB. Sepsis/septic shock: participation of the microcirculation: an abbreviated review. Crit Care Med 1996;24(6):1072–8.
51. Bateman RM, Walley KR. Microvascular resuscitation as a therapeutic goal in severe sepsis. Crit Care 2005;9(Suppl 4):S27–32.
52. Trzeciak S, Cinel I, Phillip Dellinger R, et al. Resuscitating the microcirculation in sepsis: the central role of nitric oxide, emerging concepts for novel therapies, and challenges for clinical trials. Acad Emerg Med 2008;15(5):399–413.
53. de Montmollin E, Annane D. Year in review 2010: critical care–multiple organ dysfunction and sepsis. Crit Care 2011;15(6):236.
54. De Backer D, Ortiz JA, Salgado D. Coupling microcirculation to systemic hemodynamics. Curr Opin Crit Care 2010;16(3):250–4.
55. Croner RS, Hoerer E, Kulu Y, et al. Hepatic platelet and leukocyte adherence during endotoxemia. Crit Care 2006;10(1):R15.
56. Marechal X, Favory R, Joulin O, et al. Endothelial glycocalyx damage during endotoxemia coincides with microcirculatory dysfunction and vascular oxidative stress. Shock 2008;29(5):572–6.
57. Cabrales P, Vazquez BY, Tsai AG, et al. Microvascular and capillary perfusion following glycocalyx degradation. J Appl Phys (1985) 2007;102(6):2251–9.
58. Nelson A, Berkestedt I, Schmidtchen A, et al. Increased levels of glycosaminoglycans during septic shock: relation to mortality and the antibacterial actions of plasma. Shock 2008;30(6):623–7.
59. Lidington D, Ouellette Y, Li F, et al. Conducted vasoconstriction is reduced in a mouse model of sepsis. J Vasc Res 2003;40(2):149–58.
60. Tyml K, Wang X, Lidington D, et al. Lipopolysaccharide reduces intercellular coupling in vitro and arteriolar conducted response in vivo. Am J Physiol Heart Circ Physiol 2001;281(3):H1397–406.
61. Ellsworth ML, Liu A, Dawant B, et al. Analysis of vascular pattern and dimensions in arteriolar networks of the retractor muscle in young hamsters. Microvasc Res 1987;34(2):168–83.
62. Palmer RM, Ferrige AG, Moncada S. Nitric oxide release accounts for the biological activity of endothelium-derived relaxing factor. Nature 1987;327(6122):524–6.
63. Cunha FQ, Assreuy J, Moss DW, et al. Differential induction of nitric oxide synthase in various organs of the mouse during endotoxaemia: role of TNF-alpha and IL-1-beta. Immunology 1994;81(2):211–5.
64. Baskurt OK, Temiz A, Meiselman HJ. Red blood cell aggregation in experimental sepsis. J Lab Clin Med 1997;130(2):183–90.
65. Morin MJ, Unno N, Hodin RA, et al. Differential expression of inducible nitric oxide synthase messenger RNA along the longitudinal and crypt-villus axes of the intestine in endotoxemic rats. Crit Care Med 1998;26(7):1258–64.

66. Revelly JP, Ayuse T, Brienza N, et al. Endotoxic shock alters distribution of blood flow within the intestinal wall. Crit Care Med 1996;24(8):1345–51.
67. Lam C, Tyml K, Martin C, et al. Microvascular perfusion is impaired in a rat model of normotensive sepsis. J Clin Invest 1994;94(5):2077–83.
68. Farquhar I, Martin CM, Lam C, et al. Decreased capillary density in vivo in bowel mucosa of rats with normotensive sepsis. J Surg Res 1996;61(1):190–6.
69. Lundy DJ, Trzeciak S. Microcirculatory dysfunction in sepsis. Crit Care Nurs Clin North Am 2011;23(1):67–77.
70. Baskurt OK, Gelmont D, Meiselman HJ. Red blood cell deformability in sepsis. Am J Respir Crit Care Med 1998;157(2):421–7.
71. Eichelbronner O, Sielenkamper A, Cepinskas G, et al. Endotoxin promotes adhesion of human erythrocytes to human vascular endothelial cells under conditions of flow. Crit Care Med 2000;28(6):1865–70.
72. Groom AC, Ellis CG, Wrigley SJ, et al. Capillary network morphology and capillary flow. Int J Microcirc Clin Exp 1995;15(5):223–30.
73. Kirschenbaum LA, McKevitt D, Rullan M, et al. Importance of platelets and fibrinogen in neutrophil-endothelial cell interactions in septic shock. Crit Care Med 2004;32(9):1904–9.
74. Secor D, Li F, Ellis CG, et al. Impaired microvascular perfusion in sepsis requires activated coagulation and P-selectin-mediated platelet adhesion in capillaries. Intensive Care Med 2010;36(11):1928–34.
75. Moreau D, Timsit JF, Vesin A, et al. Platelet count decline: an early prognostic marker in critically ill patients with prolonged ICU stays. Chest 2007;131(6):1735–41.
76. Di Giantomasso D, May CN, Bellomo R. Vital organ blood flow during hyperdynamic sepsis. Chest 2003;124(3):1053–9.
77. McCuskey RS, Urbaschek R, Urbaschek B. The microcirculation during endotoxemia. Cardiovasc Res 1996;32(4):752–63.
78. Spronk PE, Ince C, Gardien MJ, et al. Nitroglycerin in septic shock after intravascular volume resuscitation. Lancet 2002;360(9343):1395–6.
79. De Backer D, Creteur J, Preiser JC, et al. Microvascular blood flow is altered in patients with sepsis. Am J Respir Crit Care Med 2002;166(1):98–104.
80. Ellis CG, Bateman RM, Sharpe MD, et al. Effect of a maldistribution of microvascular blood flow on capillary O(2) extraction in sepsis. Am J Physiol Heart Circ Physiol 2002;282(1):H156–64.
81. Legrand M, Bezemer R, Kandil A, et al. The role of renal hypoperfusion in development of renal microcirculatory dysfunction in endotoxemic rats. Intensive Care Med 2011;37(9):1534–42.
82. Walley KR. Heterogeneity of oxygen delivery impairs oxygen extraction by peripheral tissues: theory. J Appl Phys (1985) 1996;81(2):885–94.
83. Goldman D, Bateman RM, Ellis CG. Effect of decreased O2 supply on skeletal muscle oxygenation and O2 consumption during sepsis: role of heterogeneous capillary spacing and blood flow. Am J Physiol Heart Circ Physiol 2006;290(6):H2277–85.
84. Humer MF, Phang PT, Friesen BP, et al. Heterogeneity of gut capillary transit times and impaired gut oxygen extraction in endotoxemic pigs. J Appl Phys (1985) 1996;81(2):895–904.
85. Cunnion RE, Schaer GL, Parker MM, et al. The coronary circulation in human septic shock. Circulation 1986;73(4):637–44.
86. Dhainaut JF, Huyghebaert MF, Monsallier JF, et al. Coronary hemodynamics and myocardial metabolism of lactate, free fatty acids, glucose, and ketones in patients with septic shock. Circulation 1987;75(3):533–41.

87. Kreymann G, Grosser S, Buggisch P, et al. Oxygen consumption and resting metabolic rate in sepsis, sepsis syndrome, and septic shock. Crit Care Med 1993;21(7):1012–9.
88. Brealey D, Brand M, Hargreaves I, et al. Association between mitochondrial dysfunction and severity and outcome of septic shock. Lancet 2002; 360(9328):219–23.
89. Schumacker PT, Samsel RW. Oxygen delivery and uptake by peripheral tissues: physiology and pathophysiology. Crit Care Clin 1989;5(2):255–69.
90. Simonson SG, Welty-Wolf K, Huang YT, et al. Altered mitochondrial redox responses in gram negative septic shock in primates. Circ Shock 1994;43(1): 34–43.
91. Boekstegers P, Weidenhofer S, Pilz G, et al. Peripheral oxygen availability within skeletal muscle in sepsis and septic shock: comparison to limited infection and cardiogenic shock. Infection 1991;19(5):317–23.
92. Manthous CA, Schumacker PT, Pohlman A, et al. Absence of supply dependence of oxygen consumption in patients with septic shock. J Crit Care 1993; 8(4):203–11.
93. Goedhart PT, Khalilzada M, Bezemer R, et al. Sidestream Dark Field (SDF) imaging: a novel stroboscopic LED ring-based imaging modality for clinical assessment of the microcirculation. Opt Express 2007;15(23):15101–14.
94. Donati A, Damiani E, Luchetti MM, et al. Microcirculatory effects of the transfusion of leukodepleted or non-leukodepleted red blood cells in septic patients: a pilot study. Crit Care 2014;18(1):R33.

Vasopressor Weaning in Patients with Septic Shock

Daniel L. Arellano, MSN, RN, ACNP-BC, CCRN, CEN[a,b,*],
Sandra K. Hanneman, PhD, RN, FAAN[c]

KEYWORDS

- Sepsis • Septic shock • Vasopressor • Titration • Wean • Hypotension

KEY POINTS

- The authors recommend close monitoring and aggressive titration of vasopressors to maximize both vasopressor treatment and weaning in patients with sepsis.
- The rationale for mean arterial pressure (MAP) greater than or equal to 65 mm Hg is based on the physiologic concept of autoregulation of blood flow, the body's attempt to withhold or divert blood flow to the most critical organs.
- Close monitoring includes narrow alarm parameters for MAP and heart rate to minimize adverse events and facilitate rapid attainment of MAP greater than or equal to 65 mm Hg and subsequent discontinuance of vasopressor therapy.
- Implementation of a weaning protocol inclusive of narrow monitor alarm parameters will decrease the total time and dose of vasopressor therapy, thereby ensuring adequate tissue perfusion with minimal adverse events.

INTRODUCTION

Sepsis is the leading cause of death in noncoronary intensive care units (ICUs) in the United States[1] and the 11th leading cause of death overall.[2,3] More than 750,000 cases of severe sepsis occur annually.[2] Septic shock, defined as the presence of an infection that causes organ dysfunction and adverse hemodynamic changes,[1] results from severe sepsis. This condition carries a mortality rate of 50% to 70% in the ICU setting.[1] Causes of death are multifactorial, but there is strong evidence to

Disclosures: D. Arellano is a PhD student at the University of Texas Health Science Center at Houston. His dissertation chair is S.K. Hanneman. He holds a scholarship from PARTNERS at the University of Texas Health Science Center at Houston School of Nursing.
[a] Division of Critical Care, Department of Medicine, Houston Methodist Hospital, 6550 Fannin Street, Suite SM1001, Houston, TX 77030, USA; [b] Department of Family Health, School of Nursing, University of Texas Health Science Center at Houston, Room# 796, 6901 Bertner Avenue, Houston, TX 77030, USA; [c] Center for Nursing Research, School of Nursing, University of Texas Health Science Center at Houston, Room #594, 6901 Bertner Avenue, Houston, TX 77030, USA
* Corresponding author. Department of Family Health, School of Nursing, University of Texas Health Science Center at Houston, Room# 796, 6901 Bertner Avenue, Houston, TX 77030.
E-mail address: Daniel.L.Arellano@uth.tmc.edu

suggest that the use of vasopressors contributes to complications and overall mortality. Complications associated with vasopressor use include myocardial and splanchnic ischemia.[4,5] Despite the dangerous complications associated with these drugs, the use of vasopressors for sepsis-induced hypotension is critical to maintain adequate blood pressure and tissue perfusion after fluid resuscitation efforts have failed. This article aims to discuss the pathophysiology of sepsis and hypotension, briefly review current guidelines for treating sepsis, detail the pharmacologic actions of vasopressor therapy, and provide literature and discussion to support rapid downward titration of these drugs with close patient monitoring.

PATHOPHYSIOLOGY OF SEPSIS AND HYPOTENSION

The pathophysiology of sepsis informs assessment and treatment decisions. When a bacterial pathogen enters the sterile environment of the body, the inflammatory response is invoked with the release of neutrophils and later macrophages to promote bacterial phagocytosis. These leukocytes release proinflammatory and antiinflammatory mediators to facilitate phagocytosis. Such proinflammatory cytokines as tumor necrosis factor-alpha (TNF-α) and interleukin-1 (IL-1) cause fever, activate coagulation, and increase endothelial permeability to recruit additional macrophages for suppression of bacterial growth.[6] Such antiinflammatory cytokines as IL-10 and IL-1 receptor antagonist also are released to counter the massive inflammatory response and promote homeostasis.[6] If these mechanisms are able to balance each other appropriately, the infectious process is eliminated and tissue repair and healing can occur. However, if the proinflammatory cytokines extend their reach beyond the area of infection, a generalized systemic response is manifested.

Transition from infection to sepsis occurs (**Fig. 1**) when large quantities of proinflammatory cytokines are released into the bloodstream. In addition to leukocytosis, fever, and activation of coagulation and fibrinolysis, TNF-α and IL-1 promote hypotension.[6] The complement plasma protein system is activated to clear the bacterial components from the blood stream. Subsequent antigen-antibody complexes form large proteins that damage the tissues, and low circulating T- and B-lymphocytes contribute to the immunosuppression seen during sepsis.[7] Tissue ischemia develops when microcirculatory lesions formed during the activation of coagulation reduce oxygen delivery. Subsequent endothelial damage triggers the release of reactive oxygen species, lytic enzymes, and such vasoactive substances as nitric oxide.[6] Endotoxin released from bacterial cell walls, TNF-α, and nitric oxide all destroy the mitochondrial matrix within the cell, resulting in cell injury, reduced energy metabolism, and decreased oxygen utilization.[6] Impaired utilization of oxygen causes organ failure in sepsis. Proinflammatory cytokines delay macrophage apoptosis, which prolongs the inflammatory response and increases ischemia and organ failure. Because the cellular injury affects every organ system, patients experience renal, myocardial, pulmonary, hepatic, and nervous system failure.[6]

Nitric oxide release secondary to endothelial damage and endotoxin is the major contributor to hypotension in septic shock because nitric oxide is a potent vasodilator. If vasodilatation is not treated rapidly, cardiac failure may result and lead to further tissue hypoperfusion and multisystem organ failure.[8] The increased endothelial permeability from proinflammatory cytokines causes vascular leakage and hypovolemia.[6]

TREATMENT GUIDELINES FOR SEPSIS

Monitoring tissue perfusion is a key guideline of the Surviving Sepsis Campaign[1] to prevent, assess, and treat rapid deterioration of patient condition. Systematically

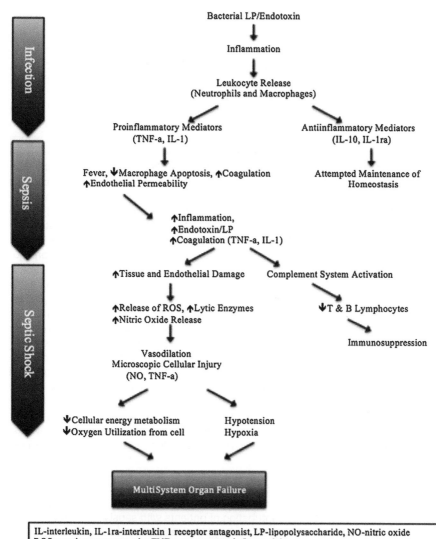

Fig. 1. Pathophysiology of septic shock.

IL-interleukin, IL-1ra-interleukin 1 receptor antagonist, LP-lipopolysaccharide, NO-nitric oxide ROS-reactive oxygen species, TNF-a-tumor necrosis factor-alpha,

addressing all of the mechanisms causing reduced tissue perfusion in septic shock can improve patient condition. Detailed guidelines for doing so have been provided by various entities.

Two important sources that health care providers use for the management of sepsis are the Surviving Sepsis Campaign[1] and the Early Goal-Directed Therapy (EGDT) Collaborative Group.[9] Recommendations of the Surviving Sepsis Campaign likely are the most familiar to those who work in the ICU. Providers who work in the emergency department or smaller institutions may also use recommendations provided by the EGDT Collaborative Group.

Surviving Sepsis Campaign Guidelines

The Surviving Sepsis Campaign was initiated in 2004, with periodic updates to the guidelines; the most recent update was in 2012.[1] The recommendations are extensive, and a comprehensive review is encouraged for all who work in the ICU; however, consistent with the focus of this *Clinics* issue on tissue perfusion and oxygenation, only the relevant guidelines are discussed here.

The guidelines emphasize early recognition and management of sepsis. Evidence has shown better outcomes if sepsis identification and treatment is started within 6 hours of the onset of illness. Hypotension should be managed initially with a 30 mL/kg bolus of intravenous crystalloid therapy to maintain mean arterial pressure (MAP) greater than or equal to 65 mm Hg. If crystalloid therapy is unsuccessful, colloids are infused. The guidelines recommend albumin over hetastarch because renal complications are less severe after administration of albumin compared with hetastarch.[1] The goals of fluid resuscitation include central venous pressure (CVP) of 8 to 12 mm Hg, MAP greater than or equal to 65 mm Hg, urine output (UO) greater than or equal to 0.5 mL/kg/h, and venous oxygen saturation of 65% to 70%. If fluid resuscitation efforts fail to establish MAP greater than or equal to 65 mm Hg, vasopressor therapy is indicated.[1]

Norepinephrine is the vasopressor recommended for initial use by the Surviving Sepsis Campaign because the alpha-1 and trace beta-1 effects of this vasopressor are the best mechanisms of action to achieve hemodynamic stability in the pathologic context of sepsis. A primary mechanism of septic shock is vasodilation from the release of nitric oxide, and direct stimulation of alpha-1 receptors promotes constriction of the vasculature. If norepinephrine therapy is ineffective, the addition of epinephrine is recommended. Vasopressin can be added to this therapy combination in an effort to replete the body's natural vasopressin stores. Vasopressin should not be used as the initial vasopressor; it is only used to augment the endogenous release of arginine vasopressin (ie, antidiuretic hormone) from the posterior pituitary gland, thereby increasing water retention. The guidelines recommend placement of arterial and central catheters to ensure accurate, precise, and timely measurement and monitoring of hemodynamic variables.

The Surviving Sepsis guidelines also address efforts to improve cardiac output and oxygenation. Dobutamine therapy is used to improve cardiac output and reduce filling pressures in the heart. A hemoglobin level of 7 to 9 g/dL is targeted to ensure adequate delivery of oxygen to the tissues. Intubation of patients with sepsis is common due to hemodynamic instability, administration of aggressive fluid resuscitation, and/or presence of a septic source within the lungs. Application of evidence-based treatment of acute respiratory distress syndrome is also recommended, which includes the aggressive use of positive end-expiratory pressure to improve alveolar-arterial oxygen exchange. Monitoring oxygenation and ventilation with the use of mixed venous or central venous oxygen saturation levels is indicated, as well as arterial blood gas surveillance. Overall, the Surviving Sepsis Campaign guidelines offer the most comprehensive recommendations for the diagnosis, management, and monitoring of patients with sepsis and septic shock.

Early Goal-directed Therapy

The Early Goal-directed Therapy (EGDT) Collaborative Group was established before the development of the Surviving Sepsis guidelines. The research conducted by this group was important to the establishment of guidelines for the management of patients with sepsis.[9] The main goal of the primary study was to evaluate the use of

EGDT in the initial 6 hours of sepsis for patients in the emergency department. The monitoring of these patients extended beyond the standard therapy and remains a critical guideline that continues to be implemented in practice today.

Similar to the Surviving Sepsis guidelines, EGDT emphasizes early recognition of patients with sepsis. Targeted resuscitation begins with frequent vital sign, laboratory data, and cardiac and pulse oximetry monitoring. Urinary, arterial, and central venous catheterizations are recommended. Monitoring of central venous oxygen saturation (ScVO$_2$) is a core EGDT guideline.[1] ScVO$_2$ is a direct measurement of the oxygen saturation of blood returning to the heart, and values reflect the relation between oxygen delivery to the tissues and oxygen consumption.[10] The EGDT Collaborative Group recommends maintaining ScVO$_2$ greater than or equal to 70%, and, as with the Surviving Sepsis Campaign, targeting CVP 8 to 12 mm Hg, MAP greater than or equal to 65 mm Hg, and UO greater than or equal to 0.5 mL/kg/h. EGDT interventions also include the maintenance of arterial oxygen saturation greater than 93% with supplemental oxygen therapy and/or intubation if needed.[9] Hematocrit should be maintained at greater than 30% to improve oxygen delivery to the tissues. No recommendations were made for specific vasopressor therapies or inotropic agents.[9] The EGDT guidelines do not differ much from those of the Surviving Sepsis Campaign; however, it is noted that the hallmark EGDT recommendation is the rapid and early introduction of monitoring even when the patient is in the emergency department. The EGDT approach to sepsis management has been shown to significantly improve mortality outcomes in patients with sepsis.[9]

AUTOREGULATION OF BLOOD FLOW

The 2 guidelines discussed earlier recommend the titration of therapies in patients with sepsis to an MAP greater than or equal to 65 mm Hg. The rationale for MAP greater than or equal to 65 mm Hg is based on the physiologic concept of autoregulation of blood flow, that is, the body's attempts to withhold or divert blood flow to the most critical organs (ie, brain, heart, and kidneys),[11] whereas, the overall concept of autoregulation is dated, well validated, and described in the literature. The autoregulation of blood flow mechanism is described as protective. At MAP less than 65 mm Hg, the body is unable to divert blood flow from the less important to the most critical organs. When MAP is less than 65 mm Hg, organ perfusion becomes dependent solely on pressure, and autoregulatory mechanisms are deactivated. If MAP climbs too high (eg, MAP >120 mm Hg), blood is diverted away from organs to prevent the pressure within the arteries from causing subsequent rupture or other damage.[11]

VASOPRESSORS USED IN THE MANAGEMENT OF SEPTIC SHOCK

Vasopressor therapy is an integral component of hemodynamic management in patients with sepsis and septic shock. The therapy is recommended by every major guideline when fluid resuscitation interventions fail to increase MAP greater than or equal to 65 mm Hg. The 5 vasopressors addressed in this article are norepinephrine, epinephrine, dopamine, vasopressin, and phenylephrine. Such drugs as dobutamine and milrinone are excluded because they are classified as inotropes and therefore can decrease systemic blood pressure because of their vasodilatory effects. Each of the 5 vasopressors stimulates specific receptor sites and has a different mechanism of action. The authors address vasopressor receptors in the later discussion and review the application of each vasopressor in the treatment of septic shock.

Receptors

Vasopressors increase blood pressure through the stimulation of alpha-1, beta-1, dopamine, and vasopressin receptors. *Alpha-1* receptors are mainly involved with smooth muscle contraction. Alpha-adrenoceptor agonists (α-agonists) stimulate the Gq protein that activates smooth muscle contraction through the inositol triphosphate signal transduction pathway.[12] Stimulation of these receptors induces vasoconstriction within the periphery and visceral organs, which mimics the effects of sympathetic adrenergic nerve activation of the blood vessels. Beta-adrenoceptors/beta agonists activate adenylyl cyclase to form cyclic adenosine monophosphate (cAMP) from adenosine triphosphate.[12] Through complex pathways, high levels of cAMP cause increased calcium entry into the cells, which heightens cardiac contractility (inotropy).[12] Beta-adrenoceptors also stimulate the opening of ion channels in the heart that promotes electrical current through the sinoatrial node (chronotropy).[12] *Beta-1* receptors increase cardiac output by increasing the heart rate and stroke volume; however, they have no direct action on the vasculature.

Dopamine receptors are unique in how they contribute to increasing the blood pressure in septic shock. Dopamine agonists (such as intravenous dopamine) activate dopamine receptors that cause vasodilation in the vasculature throughout the body and particularly within the kidneys.[13] However, the actions of dopamine agonists are dose-dependent. Administration of low-dose intravenous dopamine (1–5 mcg/kg/min) stimulates vasodilation in the small vessels and within the kidneys. Moderate doses act as a precursor to norepinephrine synthesis and stimulate norepinephrine release, which activates alpha-1 and beta-1 receptors. Doses ranging from 5 to 10 mcg/kg/min promote effects similar to beta-1 stimulation, including increased heart rate and stroke volume. High doses (10–20 mcg/kg/min) cause alpha-1 effects and profound vasoconstriction, thereby increasing the blood pressure.[13]

There are 2 different *vasopressin* receptors. Vasopressin-1 is stimulated by release of arginine vasopressin and acts on vascular smooth muscle. Stimulation causes profound vasoconstriction due to an increase in intracellular calcium.[12] Vasopressin-2 also is stimulated by the release of arginine vasopressin, but it acts on the kidneys to retain more water. The primary mechanism of vasoconstriction from vasopressin is from the stimulation of vasopressin-1 receptors.[12] Receptor mechanisms of action have implications for the complications associated with vasopressor therapy (**Table 1**).

Vasopressors

Norepinephrine is recommended as the first drug to treat hypotension during septic shock.[1] It primarily stimulates alpha-1 receptors (which counteracts the vasodilatation process), but does mildly stimulate beta-1 (see **Table 1**).[12] Norepinephrine has been shown to significantly increase MAP with only small changes in heart rate and cardiac output, leading to higher systemic vascular resistance.[14,15] There has been some concern in the clinical setting about the vasoconstrictive properties of norepinephrine on renal perfusion; however, norepinephrine actually increases renal blood flow by providing a higher perfusion pressure and thus increases glomerular filtration.[16]

Epinephrine is the second drug of choice in treating a patient with sepsis-induced hypotension.[1] At low doses it primarily stimulates beta-1 receptors that increase cardiac contractility. At high doses, alpha-1 receptors become activated and respond similarly to norepinephrine with profound vasoconstriction. Complications associated with this drug, like with norepinephrine, include arrhythmias and ischemia (see **Table 1**).

Vasopressin is the third drug of choice for treating a patient with sepsis-induced hypotension.[1] It is indicated for use in patients who have been septic for more than

Table 1
Common vasopressors used in the ICU setting for hypotension associated with septic shock

Vasopressor	Usual Dose Range	Receptor Affinity	Side Effects	Titration Recommendation
Norepinephrine	0.5–30 mcg/min 0.01–3 mcg/kg/min	$\alpha 1$ and $\beta 1$ $\alpha 1 > \beta 1$	Tachycardia, arrhythmias, cardiac and tissue ischemia	2–5 mcg/min every 3–5 min
Epinephrine	0.5–10 mcg/min 0.01–1 mcg/kg/min	$\beta 1 > \alpha 1$ Low doses = β High doses = α	Tachycardia, arrhythmias, cardiac and tissue ischemia	0.5–2 mcg/min every 3–5 min
Vasopressin	0.01–0.1 U/min (fixed dose 0.04 U/min)	V1 Receptors	Arrhythmias, cardiac, tissue, visceral, and splanchnic ischemia	0.01 U/min every 10–15 min
Dopamine	2–20 mcg/kg/min	DA = <5 mcg/kg/min $\beta 1$ = 5–10 mcg/kg/min $\alpha 1$ = 10–20 mcg/kg/min	Tachycardia, arrhythmias, cardiac and tissue ischemia	2–5 mcg/kg/min every 5–10 min
Phenylephrine	10–200 mcg/min	Pure $\alpha 1$	Reflex bradycardia, tissue and visceral ischemia	10–20 mcg/min every 3–5 min

24 hours, wherein vasopressin deficiency is presumed.[17] To compensate for the deficiency, vasopressin is administered at a fixed rate of 0.04 U/min.[17] As discussed earlier, vasopressin has an affinity for vasopressin-1 receptors and acts as a powerful vasoconstrictor.

Dopamine is cautiously recommended for use in patients with sepsis. Recall that dopamine is a dose-dependent vasopressor. For therapeutic use in sepsis, doses range from moderate to high and act primarily on beta-1 and alpha-1 receptors. Therefore, dopamine increases cardiac contractility and stroke volume and, with higher doses, causes vasoconstriction. A higher incidence of such complications as cardiac arrhythmias, altered hormone regulation, and decreased splanchnic perfusion preclude the routine use of dopamine in septic shock.

Phenylephrine is the last drug recommended for use in hypotension secondary to septic shock. This vasopressor is used to stimulate purely alpha-1 receptors. It is only recommended for use in a select group of patients with septic shock. This group includes those with serious arrhythmias from other vasopressors, salvage therapy when other vasopressors are ineffective, or in situations of known high-output heart failure. The side effects of reflex bradycardia (from the stimulation of baroreceptors by increased blood pressure); tissue ischemia in the periphery, heart, and visceral organs; and decreased cardiac output secondary to increased systemic vascular resistance increase the workload of the heart and lower overall outflow of blood, thereby reducing oxygen delivery to the tissues.[1,12]

Dosing of vasopressors to target a specific MAP is often a point of contention.[18,19] Each unit, hospital, or institution has guidelines for administration of the vasopressors most commonly used in the particular setting. Nonetheless, there is general consensus on standard dosing of these drugs (see Table 1) to maintain MAP greater than or equal to 65 mm Hg.[1] The typical order for the addition of vasopressors as recommended in clinical guidelines[1] for the patient in septic shock is (1) norepinephrine, (2) epinephrine, (3) vasopressin, (4) dopamine, and (5) phenylephrine (Fig. 2). Of course, escalation and weaning of therapy is gauged by patient condition and MAP.

Because the complications of vasopressor therapy are serious and potentially lethal, health care providers need to closely monitor patients, keep the drugs within the recommended ranges, and wean patients off of the vasopressor as soon as feasible.

VASOPRESSOR WEANING
Prioritization of Vasopressor Weaning

When the patient is hemodynamically stable with a therapeutic MAP and after a thorough assessment of perfusion status has been completed (mentation, UO, etc.) vasopressor weaning should commence. Although the best way to wean vasopressors is controversial,[18] general principles should be followed. Table 1 provides the most common weaning dosages for each drug as well as the time interval for further titration. It is important to note that patients with baseline hypertension often perfuse better at higher pressures and may require a higher MAP to attain baseline autoregulation; this should be included in the assessment process when deciding to wean vasopressor therapy as recommended by the Surviving Sepsis Campaign. However, for those patients who are receiving several different vasopressors the question most frequently asked is which drug should be weaned first?

One consideration in determining which vasopressor to wean first is the adverse effects associated with the use of one particular drug over the other. For example, if a patient with septic shock is experiencing tachycardia and arrhythmias while on norepinephrine and phenylephrine, the recommendation is to wean the norepinephrine first

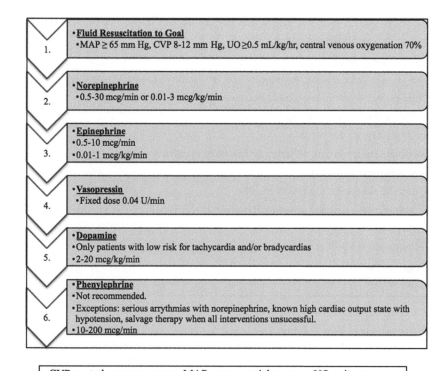

1. • **Fluid Resuscitation to Goal**
   • MAP ≥ 65 mm Hg, CVP 8-12 mm Hg, UO ≥0.5 mL/kg/hr, central venous oxygenation 70%

2. • **Norepinephrine**
   • 0.5-30 mcg/min or 0.01-3 mcg/kg/min

3. • **Epinephrine**
   • 0.5-10 mcg/min
   • 0.01-1 mcg/kg/min

4. • **Vasopressin**
   • Fixed dose 0.04 U/min

5. • **Dopamine**
   • Only patients with low risk for tachycardia and/or bradycardias
   • 2-20 mcg/kg/min

6. • **Phenylephrine**
   • Not recommended.
   • Exceptions: serious arrythmias with norepinephrine, known high cardiac output state with hypotension, salvage therapy when all interventions unsuccessful.
   • 10-200 mcg/min

CVP-central venous pressure. MAP-mean arterial pressure. UO-urine output

Fig. 2. Algorithm for treating hypotension in septic shock.

to reduce the occurrence of tachycardia and dysrhythmias.[1] If the patient is experiencing reduced cardiac output on dopamine and phenylephrine, the recommendation is to wean the phenylephrine before dopamine because phenylephrine decreases, whereas dopamine increases cardiac output.[20]

Another factor to consider is the first-line drug of choice used to treat hypotension in patients with septic shock. If, for example, the patient is on vasopressin, phenylephrine, and norepinephrine, and is ready to wean off vasopressor therapy, he or she should be weaned off the phenylephrine, followed by vasopressin, because norepinephrine is the drug of choice for sepsis-induced hypotension.

A third factor to consider is the individual patient's response to different vasopressors, which involves clinical judgment. A given patient may respond better to one particular vasopressor than others. For example, a patient may show marked improvement in MAP after the addition of dopamine to the standard norepinephrine regimen. In such a case, the clinician would wean the norepinephrine first to allow the drug that elicits the best response to remain in use longer. There is no guideline substitute for clinical judgment, and the best drug for a given patient should be used to maintain hemodynamic status.

Weaning Prototype

No standardized weaning recommendations are provided by the major guidelines, and research on vasopressor weaning methods is limited. Instead, vasopressor weaning is guided by patient response to drug titration and clinical nursing judgment. It is therefore important to use a systematic method for weaning vasopressors. **Box 1** provides a

---

Box 1
Prototype for vasopressor weaning[a]

1. Patient maintaining stable hemodynamics and adequately fluid resuscitated
2. Determine priority of vasopressor weaning and/or collaborate with provider
3. Change monitor alarms to promote rapid weaning
   - MAP goal (eg, 65–70 mm Hg)
   - HR goal (eg, 80–120 BPM)
4. Wean vasopressors based on **Table 1** or hospital/unit policy
5. Closely monitor perfusion
   - Other vital signs: O_2 saturation, HR, RR
   - Central venous oxygen saturation (if present)
   - UO
6. Discontinue vasopressors

[a] Patient specific.
Abbreviations: BPM, beats per minute; HR, heart rate; O_2, oxygen.

---

prototype for systematic vasopressor weaning. Erratic changes in blood pressure during vasopressor titration can be detrimental to patient outcome and prolong weaning.

The prototype for vasopressor weaning in septic shock includes several steps. First and foremost, ensure the patient has stable hemodynamics and has been adequately resuscitated with fluids. Weaning should commence when blood pressure readings are consistently above the MAP goal at rest and after a thorough assessment of perfusion status has been completed. Secondly, determine which vasopressor should be weaned first if the patient is receiving more than one; this decision might be made collaboratively with the treatment provider and team. Third, change the monitor alarms to narrow weaning parameters to enhance aggressiveness of titration. For example, an upper MAP alarm of 70 mm Hg would trigger downward titration more rapidly than one set at 90 mm Hg. Fourth, utilization of standardized dosing during the titration process (see **Table 1**) will help to decrease erratic swings in MAP. Fifth, examination of other vital signs, central venous oxygen saturation, and UO will give the nurse a good assessment of perfusion status during titration. For example, an increase in heart rate may indicate a compensatory response to titration intolerance and suggest the need for slower titration to prevent subsequent hypotension. Finally, once vasopressor therapy has been discontinued, it is important to continue close monitoring of the patient's hemodynamics and indicators of perfusion status (mentation, UO, $ScVO_2$, etc.) in case therapy needs to be resumed. Using narrow alarm parameters even after the vasopressors have been discontinued can help prevent adverse outcomes.

OPTIMAL MONITORING OF PATIENTS WITH VASOPRESSOR THERAPY

The authors recommend close monitoring and aggressive titration to maximize both treatment and weaning of vasopressor therapy in patients with sepsis. Close monitoring includes narrow alarm parameters for MAP and heart rate to minimize adverse events and facilitate faster attainment of MAP greater than or equal to 65 mm Hg and subsequent discontinuance of vasopressor therapy. A safe alarm parameter for vasopressor titration is MAP of 65 to 70 mm Hg. This narrow parameter range ensures the blood pressure does not drop below the autoregulation threshold or climb too high during upward titration and acts as a trigger to stimulate the nurse to titrate these medications.

Few studies have examined the use of a stimulus to promote vasopressor weaning. One study used a special fuzzy logic device (which collected data and applied them to an algorithm) for rapid titration and demonstrated a statistically significant positive change in outcomes,[18] but it did not focus on monitor alarms. A future project could include a randomized controlled trial of patients who have narrowed monitor alarms for vasopressor titration (MAP 65–70 mm Hg) versus those who receive standard titration without the reminder of an alarm. More research is indicated to observe if patient outcomes are improved with the use of narrow alarm parameters or other stimuli for aggressive titration of vasopressor therapy.

The suggestion of MAP of 65 to 70 mm Hg as an alarm parameter is based on clinical experience, national guidelines, and the concept of autoregulation of blood flow.[11] Patients with baseline hypertension often perfuse better at higher pressures and may require a higher MAP to attain baseline autoregulation; this should be included in the assessment process when deciding to wean vasopressor therapy as recommended by the Surviving Sepsis Campaign. Precisely, how to implement aggressive vasopressor titration merits research. Some have suggested the addition of auditory and visual monitor alarms to the complex monitoring systems within the ICU. Advanced monitoring systems can produce a small light that can serve as a nonnuisance trigger to wean vasopressor therapy to the defined parameter. Recently there has been a focus on monitor alarm optimization from large organizations such as the American Association of Critical Care Nurses (AACN) and the Joint Commission. An AACN practice alert[21,22] highlights the ubiquity of monitor alarms in the modern ICU. False pulse oximetry and electrocardiogram alarms were isolated as a major contributor to alarm fatigue. In most cases, these alarms were caused by poor adherence of the pulse oximetry probe or electrocardiogram electrodes to the patient's skin. Thus, the practice recommendations focus largely on improving monitor parameters and ensuring better adherence of the devices to the patient.

The Joint Commission report[23] takes a more global approach to managing physiologic monitoring systems. Its strategies for improvement include developing a multidisciplinary team to develop protocols for alarm parameters within each hospital care area. The report also recommends taking appropriate measures to reduce the incidence of false positive alarms, including ensuring proper adherence of equipment to the patient and limiting unnecessary equipment that may create artifact in monitor signals. Further, the Joint Commission recommends that staff clarify who is responsible for responding to alarms. Ensuring that nurses in the immediate area respond to monitor alarms outside their patient assignment will help reduce the nuisance factor, which contributes to monitor fatigue. Finally, the Joint Commission recommends ensuring a culture of safety by facilitating a review process of alarm complications and providing appropriate education as needed. The recommendations provided by both AACN and the Joint Commission may help reduce the incidence of nuisance alarms in the critical care areas.[23]

NEW DIRECTIONS IN SEPSIS RESEARCH WITH IMPLICATIONS FOR VASOPRESSOR THERAPY AND TITRATION

Recent research in ICU patients used gene expression profiling to characterize sepsis subtypes related to inflammatory signaling pathways.[24] The investigators found differences between subtypes in genes that regulate the action and metabolism of drugs, including vasopressin. Validation of different gene expression profiles in patients with sepsis may lead to targeted selection, administration, and weaning of vasopressors based on sepsis subtype in the near future. Such molecular discoveries hold promise for yielding more effective treatment and reducing vasopressor complications for the individual patient with sepsis or septic shock. However, even if more personalized vasopressor therapy is realized, aggressive vasopressor titration will continue to be important for the achievement of positive patient outcomes.

There has been increased use of echocardiography in the ICU to measure perfusion and hemodynamic status[25]; variations include transesophageal echocardiography (TEE) and transthoracic echocardiography (TTE). TEE provides a clear picture of the heart for the analysis of fluid status. However, given the invasive nature of the esophageal probe, some providers have transitioned to the use of bedside TTE. The utilization of either technique provides valuable information about preload, afterload, and contractility. Recent research[26] has demonstrated the usefulness of the 72-hour indwelling TEE probe in making hemodynamic management decisions in patients with shock. Although insertion of a TEE probe is invasive, such technologies may help vasopressor weaning by providing an indication of preload and cardiac contractility.[26]

SUMMARY

The best method for weaning vasopressors is unknown, and nurses often rely on a mixture of judgment, experience, and patient condition. This article provides a foundation for the development of a systematic vasopressor weaning approach to optimize tissue perfusion and improve patient outcomes. It is important to have a clear understanding of hypotension in septic shock to allow the clinician to make informed decisions on vasopressor selection and titration. Knowledge of vasopressor side effects, doses, and titration methods helps ensure rapid weaning of these harmful drugs. Implementation of a weaning protocol inclusive of narrow monitor alarm parameters theoretically will decrease the total time and dose of vasopressor therapy. However, this theoretical supposition has not been tested adequately and must continue to look at future directions in sepsis research to help improve the care delivered to the patients.

REFERENCES

1. Dellinger RP, Levy MM, Rhodes A, et al. Surviving sepsis campaign: international guidelines for management of severe sepsis and septic shock. Intensive Care Med 2012;39(2):165–228.
2. Angus DC, Linde-Zwirble WT, Lidicker J, et al. Epidemiology of severe sepsis in the United States: analysis of incidence, outcome, and associated costs of care. Crit Care Med 2011;29:1303–10.
3. Centers for disease control and prevention. Death statistics. 2012. Available at: http://www.cdc.gov/nchs/fastats/deaths.htm. Accessed September 24, 2013.
4. Micek ST, Shah P, Hollands JM, et al. Addition of vasopressin to norepinephrine as independent predictor of mortality in patients with refractory septic shock: an observational study. Surg Infect (Larchmt) 2007;8:189–200.
5. Nygren A, Thorén A, Ricksten S. Vasopressors and intestinal mucosal perfusion after cardiac surgery: norepinephrine vs. phenylephrine. Crit Care Med 2006; 34(3):722–9.
6. Neviere R. Pathophysiology of sepsis. In: Manaker S, Sexton DJ, editors. UpToDate. Waltham (MA): UpToDate; 2013. Available at: http://www.uptodate.com/contents/pathophysiology-of-sepsis. Accessed October 1, 2013.

7. Monserrat J, de Pablo R, Diaz-Martin D, et al. Early alterations of B cells in patients with septic shock. Crit Care 2013;17(3):R105.
8. McCance KL, Huether SE. Understanding pathophysiology. 6th edition. Maryland Heights (MO): Mosby Elsevier; 2008.
9. Rivers E, Nguyen B, Havstad S, et al. Early goal-directed therapy in the treatment of severe sepsis and septic shock. N Engl J Med 2001;345(19):1368–77.
10. Marino PL. The ICU book. New York: Lippincott Williams & Wilkins; 2006.
11. Johnson PC. Autoregulation of blood flow. Circ Res 1986;59(5):483–95.
12. Klabunde RE. Normal and abnormal blood pressure (physiology, pathophysiology and treatment). Indianapolis (IN): Richard E. Klabunde (Self published); 2013.
13. Contreras F, Fouillioux C, Bolivar A, et al. Dopamine, hypertension and obesity. Int Congr Ser 2002;1237:99–107.
14. Desjars P, Pinaud M, Potel G, et al. A reappraisal of norepinephrine therapy in human septic shock. Crit Care Med 1987;15:134–7.
15. Meadows D, Edwards JD, Wilkins RG, et al. Reversal of intractable septic shock with norepinephrine therapy. Crit Care Med 1988;16:663–6.
16. Redl-Wenzl EM, Armbruster C, Edelmann G, et al. The effects of norepinephrine on hemodynamics and renal function in severe septic shock states. Intensive Care Med 1993;19:151–4.
17. Landry DW, Levin HR, Gallant EM, et al. Vasopressin deficiency contributes to the vasodilation of septic shock. Circulation 1997;95(5):1122–5.
18. Merouani M, Guignard B, Vincent F, et al. Norepinephrine weaning in septic shock patients by closed loop control based on fuzzy logic. Crit Care 2008;12:R155.
19. Reinelt H, Radermacher P, Kiefer P, et al. Impact of exogenous beta-adrenergic receptor stimulation on hepatosplanchnic oxygen kinetics and metabolic activity in septic shock. Crit Care Med 1999;27:325–31.
20. Dellinger RP. Cardiovascular management of septic shock. Crit Care Med 2003;31(3):946–55.
21. Sendelbach S, Jepsen S, AACN Evidence-Based Practice Resources Work Group. AACN practice alert: alarm management. 2013. Available at: http://www.aacn.org/wd/practice/docs/practicealerts/alarm-management-practice-alert.pdf. Accessed September 26, 2013.
22. American Association of Critical Care Nurses. No more "white noise": improving patient alarm management. 2011. Available at: http://www.aacn.org/wd/chapters/chapterdocs/00312376/websites/docs/Patient%20Alarm%20Management%20Handouts.pdf. Accessed September 26, 2013.
23. Joint Commission on Accreditation of Healthcare Organizations. Sound the Alarm: Managing Physiologic Monitoring Systems. Jt Comm Perspect 2011;11(12):6–11.
24. Maslove D, Tang B, McLean A. Identification of sepsis subtypes in critically ill adults using gene expression profiling. Crit Care 2013;16(5):R183.
25. Vieillard-Baron A, Slama M, Mayo P, et al. A pilot study on safety and clinical utility of a single-use 72-hour indwelling transesophageal echocardiography probe. Intensive Care Med 2013;39:629–35.
26. Casserly B, Read R, Levy MM. Hemodynamic monitoring in sepsis. Crit Care Nurs Clin North Am 2011;23(1):149–69.

Index

NOTE: Page numbers of article titles are in **boldface** type.

A

Arabic world, tissue perfusion and, 300–302

B

Blood, composition of, 338–339
Blood flow, in microcirculation, 317–318
Brain perfusion and oxygenation, **389–398**
    neuroimaging techniques for, adjunctive, 385
        brain tissue oxygen tension, 393–394
        cerebral microdialysis, 394
        cerebral perfusion pressure, 392
        intracranial pressure, 392
        jugular venous oxygenation, 393
        near-infrared spectroscopy, 394–395
        positron emission tomography, 395
        single-photon emission computed tomography, 395
        transcranial Doppler, 391–393
    physiology of, blood-brain barrier in, 391
        in brain injury, 391–392
        cerebral blood flow in, 390–391
        cerebral metabolism in, 389–390
            determinants of, 390–391

C

Cardiogenic shock, microcirculatory alterations in, 401
Central venous pressure, in hemodynamic monitoring, 358
Cryopreservation, of erythrocytes, 333

D

Dopamine, for septic shock, 419–420

E

Early Goal-directed Therapy, for sepsis, 416–417
Epinephrine, for septic shock, 419–430
Erythrocytes, biopreservation of, 332
        additive solutions in, 333
        cryopreservation, 333
      deformability and aggregation of in tissue perfusion, 341–342

Crit Care Nurs Clin N Am 26 (2014) 427–432
http://dx.doi.org/10.1016/S0899-5885(14)00042-2
0899-5885/14/$ – see front matter © 2014 Elsevier Inc. All rights reserved.

ccnursing.theclinics.com

Erythrocytes (*continued*)
　Hb in, 326–327
　　affinity for carbon monoxide, 329
　　as carrier and release of NO, 330
　　environment and affinity for oxygen, 329
　　methemoglobin and, 329
　Hb in and respopnse to local environment, 326–327
　metabolic functions of, 327
　in microcirculation, 327
　in oxygen transport, 326–327
　physiologic role in oxygen delivery and implications for blood storage, **325–335**
　storage of, effects on, 332
　　physiologic effects of, 331
　　RBC storage lesion from, 330–331

F

Family experience of ICU monitoring, data analysis, qualitative, Diekelmann
　phenomenological method, 382
　　quantitative, 382
　definition of high-tech, extensive monitoring, 378
　literature review of, communication to family member, 378–379
　　need for information regarding patient status and equipment being used, 379
　　needs of family, 379–380
　　perceptions of equipment, 379–380
　　situational anxiety in family members, 379
　quantitative methodology, self-report measure, 382
　　STAI anxiety scale, 381–382
　research questions in, anxiety level of family members, 385–386
　　experience of families with extensive monitoring eqipment, 385
　　information provided about equipment and patient care in high-acuity unit, 386
　　perception of information received about the monitoring equipment, 386
　situational anxiety and, cause of, 385
　study design, family group interviews in, 381
　　hermeneutic phenomenology in, 381
　　qualitative methodology in, 380–381
　study findings, coping methods, 383
　　feelings of uncertainty, 383
　　meaning of numbers on the machines, 383
　　need for education, 384
　　overwhelmed by the machines, 383
　　quantitative, 384
　study framework, adaptation to event in, 380
　　adjustment period to illness in, 380
　　perceptions of high-tech monitoring in, 380
Family members of ICU patients, experience of, **377–388**

G

Galen of Pergamon, on circulatory system, 300, 305
Greeks, on circulatory system, 299–300

H

Harvey, William, microscopic circulatory system and, 302, 305
Hemodynamics, assessment of fluid responsiveness in, passive leg raise maneuver for, 361–362
    stroke volume optimization in, 358, 360–362
  bedside assessment techniques in, bioempedance and bioreflectance, 369–370
    capnometry, 370–371
    Doppler, 365–366
    esophageal Doppler, 363–365
    exhaled CO_2 method, 370
    pulmonary artery catheter, 363
    pulse contour method, 366–369
  cardiac output assessment and, pulse contour method in, 366–369
  current and emerging noninvasive monitoring techniques, **357–375**
  noninvasive monitoring techniques and, from cardiac pressures to parameters based on blood flow, 358–359
    passive leg raise maneuver, 361–362
    stroke volume, 358–359
    stroke volume optimization, 358, 360–362
  stroke volume assessment and, echocardiogram in, 362
    esophageal Doppler in, 363–365
    pulmonary artery catheter in, 363
Hemorheology. See also Rheology.
  blood flow in, fluid mechanics and physical determinants of, 339–340
  blood viscosity in, defined, 340–341
    shear rate and, 340
    variations in, 340–341
  composition of blood and, 338–339
  description of, 339
  erythrocytes in, aggregation of, 341–342
    deformability of, 341–342
  factors in determination of microvascular blood flow, 340
  leukocytes in, in flow resistance, 345
  in microvascular hemodynamics, **337–344**
Hypovolemia, stroke volume as indicator of, 358–359
Hypovolemic shock, microcirculatory alterations in, 401–402

L

Lactate monitoring, of tissue oxygenation, 354–355
Laser Doppler flowmetry, of tissue blood flow, 351–352

M

Malpighi, Marcello, microscopic anatomy in, 303
Microcirculation, anatomy of, 312–318, 327
  capillary endothelial cell link between tissue and blood, 327–329
  composition of, 327
  Hb in, types of, 328–329
  monitors of perfusion in, near-infrared resonance spectroscopy, 348–351
  oxygen diffusion from, 327
  in response to local tissue needs, 327

Microcirculatory oxygen transport and utilization, **311–324**
    Do$_2$ and, 320–321
    fundamentals of, convective oxygen transport, 318–319
        diffusive oxygen transport, 318–319
    macrocirculation *versus* microcirculation, 321–322
    macrovascular and microvascular systems in, 312–313
    microcirculation in, arteriolar regulation in, 315–316
        arterioles in, 312–313
        blood flow in, 317–318
        capillaries in, 313–314
        capillary density in, 314–315
        endothelium in, 316
        red blood cell in, 316–317
    oxgen consumption in, Vo$_2$ and, 320–321

    N

Near infra-red resonance spectroscopy, in assessment of cerebral oxygenation, 351
    of brain perfusion and oxygenation, 394–395
    effects on, 351
    as monitor of tissue perfusion, 348–351
NO, as carrier and release of Hb in erythrocytes, 330
    and endothelium in shock sstates, 400–401
    in septic shock, 404
Norepinephrine, for septic shock, 419–430

    P

Passive leg raise maneuver, in assessment of fluid responsiveness, 361–362
Phenylephrine, for septic shock, 419–420
Platelets, role in hemostasis, 338–339
Positron emission computed tomography, of brain perfusion and oxygenation, 395
Pulmonary artery occlusive pressure, in hemodynamic monitoring, 358

    R

Red blood cells, in microcirculation, 316–317
    in relation to flow behavior, 338
Renaissance, cardiopulmonary anatomy in, 302
Rheology. *See also* Hemorheology.
    defined, 339
    principles of, deformation and shear rate, 339
        flow rate and viscosity, 339

    S

Septic shock, microcirculatory alterations in, 402
        blood, 405
        blood flow, 405
        diffusive oxygen transport, 405–406
        endothelial dysfunction, 403–404
        nitric oxide, 404
        oxygen utilization, dysoxia, 406–407

new research directions in, echocardiography and variations in ICU, 424
  gene profiling, 423–424
pathophysiology of sepsis and hypotension in, 414–415
receptors in, alpha-adrenergic, 418
  dopamine, 418
  ß-adrenergic, 418
  vasopressin, 418
treatment guidelines for sepsis, 414–415
  autoregulation of blood flow in, 417
  Early Goal-directed Therapy, 416–417
  Surviving Sepsis Campaign, 416
vasopressors for, 417
  dobutamine, 416
  dopamine, 419–420
  dosing of, 420–421
  epinephrine, 419–420
  norepinephrine, 416, 419–420
  phenylephrine, 419–420
  vasopressin, 418–420
vasopressor therapy for, monitoring of, alarm parameters of MAP in, 422–423
vasopressor weaning in, **413–425**
  prioritization of, 419–420
  prototype for, 421–422
Shock states, general principles of microvascular function and, blood and blood flow,
  capillary, 401
    endothelium and nitric oxide, 400–401
    oxygen transport, convective and diffusive, 400
  microcirculatory alterations in, **399–412**
    in cardiogenic shock, 401
    in hypovolemic shock, 401–402
    in septic shock, 402–407
Single-photon emission tomography, of brain perfusion and oxygenation, 395
Stroke volume, in hemodynamic monitoring, 358
  as indicator of hypovolemia, 358–359
Stroke volume optimization, in assessment of fluid responsiveness, 358, 360
  resuscitation algorithm for, 360–361
Surviving Sepsis Campaign treatment guidelines, dobutamine in, 416
  norepinephrine in, 416
  positive end-expiratory pressure in, 416

T

Tissue blood flow and oxygenation, emerging monitoring techniques, **345–356**
    considerations in, accuracy and precision of device, 346
      specificity of, 347
  emerging monitoring techniques in, considerations in, limitations of device, 347
  measurement in clinical practice, 346–355
  measurement of tissue oxygenation, 348–349
  monitors of extracellular environment, for lactate, 353–355
    for tissue carbon dioxide, 353
  monitors of perfusion in microcirculation, 348–353

Tissue (*continued*)
    laser Doppler flowmetry, 351–352
    near-infrared resonance spectroscopy, 348–351
    videomicroscopy, 352
  tissue carbon dioxide monitors, gastric tonometry, 353
    sublingual capnometry, 353
  tissue oxygen tension monitors, photoluminescence quenching technique, 353
Tissue perfusion, in anatomic era, 298–299
    Aarabic world, 300–302
    Galen of Pergamon, 300, 305
    Greeks, 299–300
    Marcello Malpighi, 303–304
  cardiovascular system over time and, 305
  development of modern concepts of, **297–309**
  microscopic anatomy, 303–305
  in physiology and biochemistry era, 299
    acetyl coenzyme A in, 307
    ATP in, 306–307
    cellular metabolism in, 306–308
    oxygen and hemoglobin in, 303–304
  in Renaissance, 302
  William Harvey, 302, 305

V

Vasopressin, for septic shock, 418–420
Vasopressor weaning, in patients with septic shock, **413–425.** See also Septic shock

W

White blood cells, in determination of viscosity, 338

Moving?

Make sure your subscription moves with you!

To notify us of your new address, find your **Clinics Account Number** (located on your mailing label above your name), and contact customer service at:

Email: journalscustomerservice-usa@elsevier.com

800-654-2452 (subscribers in the U.S. & Canada)
314-447-8871 (subscribers outside of the U.S. & Canada)

Fax number: 314-447-8029

Elsevier Health Sciences Division
Subscription Customer Service
3251 Riverport Lane
Maryland Heights, MO 63043

*To ensure uninterrupted delivery of your subscription, please notify us at least 4 weeks in advance of move.

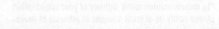